21 Medical Mysteries

By the same author:

Electrophysiological Technique

Clinical Pathology Data (2 editions and Italian translation)

Neurogenic Hypertension (2 editions)

A Computer Model of Human Respiration

Clinical Physiology (5 editions)
  With E.J.M. Campbell, J.D.H. Slater, C.R.W. Edwards and E.K. Sikora

Software for Educational Computing
  With K. Ahmed and D. Ingram

21 Medical Mysteries

JOHN DICKINSON

The Book Guild Ltd
Sussex, England

The Book Guild Ltd.
25 High Street,
Lewes, Sussex

First published 2000
© John Dickinson 2000

Set in Times
Typesetting by
Acorn Bookwork, Salisbury, Wiltshire

Printed in Great Britain by
Bookcraft (Bath) Ltd. Avon

A catalogue record for this book is
available from the British Library

ISBN 1 85776 499 4

CONTENTS

PREFACE

The object of this book is to convey some of the pleasures and excitement of scientific research – in this case research into the causes of human diseases. Although the supreme excitement may be reserved for the first discoverer, it is almost as fascinating to watch from the sidelines as nature's secrets are successively revealed. In the last 50 years there have been huge strides forward in genetics, in immunology, in epidemiology and in clinical pharmacology. There have also been innumerable smaller steps by which medical mysteries are being unravelled. Some needed new ideas or insights. Others have had to wait until a new technique allowed a previously inaccessible idea to be examined.

During a long career I have had a ringside seat watching many medical mysteries being examined and argued about. Sometimes I have entered the ring myself, with variable success. None of the fights are over. The only certainty in science is that there is no certainty about anything. But there is a lot of pleasure to be gained by gradually learning about a problem in depth. Each chapter of this book summarises a vast amount of information. I have tried to avoid oversimplifying, though it has been difficult. There is a plentiful supply of numerical data, because a rough general rule says that science begins when quantities begin to be measured. On each subject discussed here there have been hundreds, usually thousands, of relevant papers published in learned journals. It is impossible to summarise them comprehensively. But I have tried in each case first to describe the condition, disease or phenomenon as accurately and succinctly as possible, in order to set the stage for discussing the mysteries and for suggesting possible solutions to some of them.

When I was first a medical student, I wanted to find out what the mysteries were, so that I could choose the most interesting and important ones to work on when I had the chance. At that time we seemed to understand a lot. There had been marvellous advances in treatment, such as antibiotics, anti-cancer drugs and steroids. Each year since then has brought new understanding. Each has also thrown up new puzzles. Research fields get wider and wider, and more exciting, with each passing year. My choice of subjects in this book should not be taken to mean that I am not interested in the many medical mysteries

I have not discussed, but simply that those I have chosen seemed the more important and potentially soluble problems – the ones about which I had something original to say.

Since the book describes a large variety of unrelated topics, it can obviously be dipped into at random. I have tried to make it palatable to be read straight through, but more than one sitting will be needed to avoid indigestion. My last chapter, on motor neurone disease – a common, mysterious and fatal condition – is a bit different. It assumes a bit more background knowledge but I have included it to illustrate the enormous number of different lines of evidence which sometimes have to be examined by scientists trying (so far unsuccessfully in this case) to solve a particularly intractable medical mystery. For this topic I have provided a more extensive bibliography than for the other chapters. The study of motor neurone disease nicely exemplifies a universal rule of science: the more we know about a subject, the more we appreciate its complexities and realise what we don't know. But when a breakthrough comes, there is no excitement to match it.

To make the book easier for non-scientists to read I have tried to demystify all unfamiliar medical terms by giving their (usually Greek) derivations. Apart from anything else, knowing the derivation makes them easier to understand and remember. When some new unfamiliar word or concept is introduced for the first time I have defined or explained it. Later usages are cross-referenced back to the first occurrence. I hope that scientifically literate readers will not be too irritated by this, by my use of homely words like womb, by mentioning pounds, feet and inches before giving the proper SI units, or by introducing each topic in a very elementary way. All this is to allow people without much scientific training or knowledge to share some of the excitement I have felt in scientific research.

John Dickinson,
Wolfson Institute of Preventive Medicine,
St Bartholomew's & Royal London School of Medicine & Dentistry,
Charterhouse Square,
London, EC1M 6BQ.

ACKNOWLEDGEMENTS

This book could not have been written without the superb facilities I have enjoyed in the last few years at the Wolfson Institute of Preventive Medicine, which is now part of London University's medical faculty at Queen Mary and Westfield College.

I am most grateful to many kind friends and colleagues who have read or helped with individual chapters, including Eric Beck, Moran Campbell, Israel Doniach, Richard Godfrey, Jim Lawrence, Irene Leigh, Ewa Paleolog, Chris Redman, Ben Sacks, Pamela Shaw, Nick Wald, Derek Willoughby and David Wingate. Nigel Benjamin and John Swales have read the whole book. Two of our children (Mark and Caroline) have helped with several chapters. All have made useful suggestions. I am also grateful to Ian MacDonald for letting me reproduce the magnetic resonance brain scans in Chapter 3, to John Kanis for his illustrations of Paget lesions in Chapter 10, and to Cathy Driver and her colleagues in the Medical Illustration Department at Barts for preparing the other illustrations.

1

INTRODUCTION

If immortality is something to be desired, then it is achieved, as far
as humanly possible, by medical research.
(Desiderius Erasmus, 1499)[1].

Not everyone aspires to immortality, but everyone should have some
idea of what is happening today in medical research. The present rate
of discovery is speeding up tremendously as new techniques come
along to allow us to probe the human body in new ways. This book
aims to bring the reader to the threshold of knowledge about 21 fascinating but unsolved medical mysteries, most of which concern very
common conditions. Science moves fast. In another decade some of
the mysteries will be solved. Many will have become less mysterious.
On the other hand, new pathways of understanding will have opened
up. What appeared simple will have become much more complicated.
A good illustration of the increasing rate of scientific advance is shown
by what might be called the 'curve of discovery' (Fig. 1). I have
adapted this figure from one I prepared a few years ago for a
monograph on high blood pressure. The figure has a time scale which
shows the approximate dates of discovery of some 40 different factors
already known to be involved in the control of blood pressure. Any or
all of them might be involved in causing high blood pressure. The rate
of discovery shows no sign of slowing down. Since a comparable
exponential curve of discovery applies to all biological fields, this book
should just be regarded as giving a snapshot of some of today's
growing points.

All science is exciting but sometimes its scale is daunting. Astrophy-
sics deals with huge masses in space; particle physics with things so
small that their properties and very existence have to be inferred.
Molecular biology is now the fastest moving branch of biological
science, but it is difficult for anyone to understand it without a
substantial amount of factual background knowledge. It is really a
branch of anatomy – the study of how living organisms are made up.
Physiology, on the other hand – the study of how living organisms

1

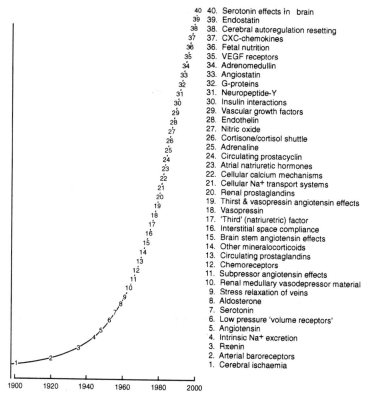

Figure 1 Historical perspective of some of the main mechanisms and systems involved in blood pressure regulation, plotted against the approximate year of their discovery.

work – is much easier for a non-specialist or even a non-scientist to understand, because the scale on which most physiology is studied is a human scale. It is also more fun. This book is about disorders of human physiology. I hope that it will convey some of the excitement of present-day science. Research needs new ideas as well as facts. We know a lot already, but there are still many gaps. All scientific research starts with asking the right questions. Sometimes the accumulation of facts alone gradually reveals the answer to a problem, but this is uncommon. Every chapter of this book asks some new questions, provides some new insights and suggests some possible answers.

My personal research interests have been mainly in disorders of the heart and circulation, especially high blood pressure. So a small part of the book is inevitably a bit autobiographical. But a look at the contents list will reveal that a wide range of topics and mysteries is

2

covered. I have personally looked after patients with every disease or condition mentioned in the book and have suggested possible explanations for some of them. Many of my suggestions will doubtless prove to be wrong, but I have tried to provide enough basic information to help others to do better. I once heard Sydney Brenner, the famous molecular biologist and a qualified medical doctor himself, make a distinction between 'scientists' and 'doctors', to the intellectual disadvantage of the latter. But a doctor who has spent his working life as a general physician, as I have, has a unique advantage over a basic scientist when it comes to thinking about medical problems. It is sometimes easier for him to think of worthwhile but unanswered questions, even though he lacks the skill and technical knowledge to solve them, because he has witnessed such an enormous variety of nature's nasty experiments – which is what diseases are.

Organisation of topics

Each chapter describes a different but fascinating medical mystery. Not all my topics can be classified as 'diseases'. The chapter on clubbing of the fingers is an intellectual exercise and a medical detective story. Many people would not classify 'chronic fatigue syndrome' (so-called 'myalgic encephalomyelitis': ME), 'irritable bowel syndrome' or even 'essential hypertension' as diseases at all. But they are certainly medical mysteries.

All the first-class scientists I have ever met have one characteristic in common: they are interested in everything. One never knows whether work in one field might not open up a completely different field. How many foresaw that ultrasound techniques would transform obstetric management? Although experienced clinicians reading this book will find their own subjects dealt with in an elementary and perhaps naive fashion, I hope that they will find some less familiar medical mysteries interesting and stimulating. I have also tried to envisage an intelligent non-scientist skimming through the book, omitting most of the technical stuff, but perhaps suddenly coming across something interesting. The technical matter and the up-to-date references at the end of the book will then allow the reader to follow right through to the latest discoveries about mechanisms.

The triumphant march of molecular biology has been one of the most spectacular advances in our understanding of disease mechanisms. The field was opened up by the characterisation of deoxyribose nucleic acid (DNA) and by the deciphering of its genetic code. There will soon be very few inherited diseases in which the responsible

3

specific genetic defects have not been identified. Cancer, which once seemed utterly mysterious, is gradually being explained in molecular terms, notably by a sequence of disadvantageous somatic mutations – some increased by damage to genes involved in DNA repair. The understanding of cancer is advancing at tremendous speed. Gene therapy for many inherited diseases is on the horizon. But there remain many important medical problems which can't be explained by single gene defects. The medical mysteries which I shall describe in this book are mostly of this kind, being partly due to environmental factors and partly due to the disadvantageous effects of many genes rather than of a single one.

2

ASTHMA: WHY IS IT INCREASING?

Asthma is a very common condition, well known to the ancient Greeks, who gave it its name. Its precise definition has been debated at many international conferences. The diagnosis implies that the asthmatic suffers from episodes in which breathing is temporarily obstructed because of narrowing of the airways of the lungs. All the airways are usually affected. The single large windpipe or trunk (the trachea) starts in the neck at the larynx. It divides in the chest into two main airways (bronchi) which lie behind the heart. Each main bronchus divides into smaller and smaller airways (bronchioles), terminating eventually in thousands of tiny air sacs (alveoli), into which inhaled air can diffuse, and thus make intimate contact with, the bloodstream. The whole structure resembles an inverted tree (Fig. 2).

The background to asthma appears always to be bronchial hyperresponsiveness, i.e. an excessive reaction by the airways to irritants such as cold air or to materials inducing 'allergy'[*]. These materials induce muscular spasm of small airways and increased secretion of sticky slime (mucus) by the linings of the larger airways. In the case of the trachea, which is a semi-rigid structure, thick mucus secretion is the cause of narrowing. In the smaller airways there is also active contraction of circular muscle in the airway walls. The internal size of the hollow tubes concerned (the 'lumen') gets smaller. A well-known relationship in physics (Poiseuille's formula) is that the resistance offered to the flow of gas or fluid through a tube increases as the fourth power of the radius. In the presence of turbulence the resistance is even higher. If, for example, the diameter of a tube through which air is flowing is halved, the resistance to airflow will increase at least 16 times. This makes for a potential trigger effect. Quite a small reduction in airway calibre can suddenly make someone feel that breathing has become difficult, a sensation technically referred to as 'dyspnoea' (the Greek word for 'bad breathing'). Lung capacity is reduced in an asthmatic attack and there is gross delay in forcefully emptying the

---

[*]'Allergy' refers to the ability of man and other animals to develop irritant or harmful responses to foreign substances after repeated exposure.

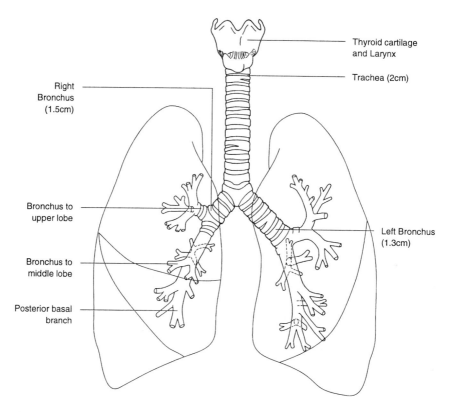

Figure 2 The main airways of the lungs, seen from the front, indicating the approximate internal diameters of the trachea and main bronchi. The two lungs are shown in outline. The left lung (on the right of the diagram) is slightly smaller than the right, because the heart occupies some of the left chest cavity.

lungs after taking a deep breath in. A simple and widely used test for airways obstruction is the 'forced expiratory volume in one second' (FEV1). An even simpler test makes use of the peak flow meter which measures the maximum speed of airflow that a subject can achieve when forcibly breathing out.

I can testify from my own experience just how suddenly breathing can get obstructed. When I was a junior doctor I had been writing down the medical details of a middle-aged woman admitted to the ward with an attack of asthma. She felt the need to pass urine, excused herself, then walked the length of the open ward. She had not returned after ten minutes or so. I assumed that she must have been constipated. Then a white-faced nurse came out and said that she had collapsed. All efforts at resuscitation were in vain. Post-mortem examination (necropsy) showed almost complete obstruction of the trachea and larger bronchi by thick tenacious mucus. It still seems hardly credible to me that someone able to talk freely and walk 40 yards could be so close to fatal asphyxia. The fact that the lavatory and bathroom area was entirely full of flowers may have provided the final trigger*. At the time, drug treatment of asthma was primitive. Steroids had not come into use. But this experience made on me an indelible impression which later I always tried to pass on to my students. Someone suffering a bad asthma attack can be living on a knife edge.

Attacks of asthma may end spontaneously, but they can be so alarming that sufferers usually start treatment by inhaling a dilating drug preparation as soon as they find that breathing has become difficult. Almost all asthmatics (999 out of 1000) improve if they regularly inhale so-called 'steroids'. This treatment is 'prophylactic' (Greek: 'pro' = before; 'phylaxis' = protection). Collectively such steroid drugs are referred to as 'glucocorticoids' because they affect the way glucose is broken down in the body. As I shall discuss later, steroids also suppress inflammation, by inhibiting the release of a gene transcription factor responsible for the local production of inflammation-promoting chemicals ('cytokines': see p. 10). Difficult breathing responsive to inhaled steroids is virtually diagnostic of asthma.

The term 'asthma' is not used for diseases of the heart or blood circulation, even though congestion of the lungs in such conditions may produce similar symptoms. 'Asthma' is also not used to describe the fixed airways obstruction which may be found in chronic bronchitis. This doesn't change suddenly and is not much helped by medical treatment. By contrast, an attack of asthma can often be relieved within minutes by the right treatment.

Epidemiology

Asthma is extremely common and getting commoner. Some estimates are of a doubling every decade. This leads to the prediction that almost everyone will have asthma in 100 years' time! At present, in Europe and in the USA, between 1% and 6% of people are affected. Over the last ten years incidence has increased by a third in the under-11s in the UK. Britain is now known as the asthma capital of Europe.

---

* Florence Nightingale – the famous and influential nurse who in 1854 transformed the treatment of wounded British soldiers in the Crimean war – had learned (correctly) that although plants produce oxygen in the light, they consume oxygen in the dark. She therefore recommended that flowers should always be taken out of hospital wards during the night. This extraordinary practice survived in the UK until about 1960!

The UK has three times the rate of Germany or Austria and 1 ½ times the rate of Ireland. In the UK more than 1000 children with asthma are admitted to hospital on most days. At any one time the prevalence has been about the same in children and adults, though young children with asthma tend to improve with time as their airways get bigger, and some people first develop the disease as adults. On average about 7% of children in Britain have asthma at some stage of their lives though its incidence may be as high as 15% in some parts of the country. Many children with episodic wheezing and probable asthma are never given that diagnosis, so the prevalence may be even greater than current estimates. Some infants develop a single episode of wheezy bronchitis due to a virus infection but never later go on to develop true asthma.

The sexes are affected about equally. There is some evidence that early childhood infections, especially measles, may protect against asthma, though early exposure to 'allergens' (things producing allergy) may be harmful. It has also been suggested that children who have often been given antibiotics to treat minor bacterial infections may thereby become more liable to asthma. The picture is confusing.

The inheritance of asthma

Asthma tends to run in families, but its inheritance is complicated. Many different genes are involved. Shared local environments may be difficult to be difficult to disentangle from genetic factors. Claims have already been made that genes localised on chromosomes* 5,6,11,12,13 and 14 are linked with asthma, but a unique 'asthma gene' has yet to be discovered. The search for it has been described as a glorious fishing expedition. It is unlikely that any single gene will prove to be

---

* The human body contains about 10^{14} (100,000,000,000,000) individual cells. Almost all cells have a nucleus containing 46 microscopic threadlike chromosomes (Greek: coloured bodies). Under the microscope each of these looks different and each has been assigned an identifying number. They are present in pairs. One of each pair comes from the individual's father, one from the mother. Chromosomes are made up of double-stranded twisted strings of DNA (deoxyribose nucleic acid). Certain sections of DNA (exons) contain a code which can be transmitted to other structures ('ribosomes') inside the cell but outside the nucleus. There the code is read and specific proteins are made. The coding sections of DNA are known as 'genes'. At present the entire sequences of genes in all the human chromosomes is being painstakingly worked out, through international collaboration. This is known as 'the human genome project'. It will gradually identify the location and eventually the chemical structure of all the (approximately) 100,000 human genes. Current predictions are that the project will be complete around 2002, or even earlier. This will make it possible to find what protein each gene codes for, thus giving clues about its possible function.

all-important. Everything suggests that the inheritance of asthma involves many different genes.

Though asthma is distressing and attacks are disabling, it is fortunately seldom fatal. Even in older people – over 55, for example – death rates from asthma in England and Wales are around 8 per year for every 100,000 people. In children the death rates are only about one twentieth of this. Even so, with the disease so common, an appreciable number of children die in an asthmatic attack each year. The summer months seem to be the worst for children, probably because of increased exposure to pollens and moulds. This contrasts with asthma deaths in the elderly, which are commoner in the winter months.

The disease is manifestly far from trivial. In the USA and some other countries asthma death rates in recent years have been rising despite widespread use of preventive medicines (prophylactics), while preventable deaths from most other causes have been steadily falling. In the UK, asthma death rates peaked in the 1960s, fell slowly in the 1970s, rose to a peak in the 1980s and are now falling again. We have really no idea why these changes occurred, though an early peak in the 1970s may have been due to overuse of inhalers with adrenaline-like drugs (see below).

Cause

The immediate precipitating cause of an attack of asthma is often exposure to an allergen – that is, to some material, usually inhaled, to which the lungs have become sensitised. Pollens and the faeces of house-dust mites are probably the commonest immediate precipitating factors. The mites live off the tiny flakes of skin that humans shed. They like a warm, damp environment to breed. When I was a student it was commonly believed that children with asthma got attacks because of emotional stress at home. This idea seemed to be confirmed because they got better when they were admitted to hospital. Now we realise that they got better mainly because beds and cots in hospitals have rubber covers and frequently-laundered cotton sheets. Both discourage house-dust mites. Prolonged avoidance of possible allergens by keeping asthmatics for several weeks in a protected hospital environment with filtered air can produce spectacular improvement in symptoms and in excessive airway reactivity[1]. This is rather strong evidence that asthma is provoked, if not actually caused, by something arriving in the air.

Asthma and 'atopy' (Greek: strangeness) are often considered

9

together, but should be considered separately. Between 15% and 50% of people in most parts of the world are atopic. This means that they react strongly and rapidly, with a large skin weal, to pinprick inoculation of many different allergens. They also have an excess of a particular class of protein antibody formerly called 'reagin' but now known as 'immunoglobulin E' or just 'IgE' in their blood. This reacts with many common allergy-inducing materials. Atopy is partly inherited and partly acquired. It is characterised by the presence of specific cytokine receptors*. The occurrence of atopy in an individual may be influenced by the time of birth, being more common in children born in the winter months, though this has yet to be confirmed. The difference probably reflects the pattern of childhood infections. Some (e.g. respiratory syncytial virus) make atopy more likely, but others (e.g. measles, hepatitis A and tuberculosis) make it less likely. Atopy has a definite association with asthma, increasing the risk of asthma about tenfold; but lots of asthmatics are not atopic. However, atopic children have been observed to be specially susceptible to air pollutants.

Do asthma treatments shed light on the cause?

The treatment of asthma is nowadays well-established and perhaps sheds some light on the possible cause. Attacks are usually treated by inhaling a 'beta-2 stimulant', a drug related to adrenaline (see below). This switches on chemical receptors in the airways. These tell the muscles in the airways to relax, thus making the air passages larger, and tell the cells lining the airways to stop producing mucus. All this makes it easier to get air in and out. Some people find that strenuous exercise starts off an attack. This may be just because breathing is stepped up, but perhaps a rush of cold air constricts the lung air passages. Many people find that inhaling a beta-2 stimulant before exercise prevents an attack. Incidentally, the opposite effect is produced by 'beta-blockers', drugs in common use for treating high blood pressure and angina. These tend to make the air passages in the lungs narrower. Such drugs are not given to asthmatics.

---

* 'Cytokines' (Greek: 'cyto' = hollow/cell; 'kine' = movement) are chemicals (technically 'polypeptides': see p. 85) which are secreted by a cell and which can diffuse to another cell and excite reactions there, after combining with a specific 'receptor'. A receptor is a chemical which is embedded in the outer membrane of a cell, but has parts of its molecule projecting inwards as well as outwards. This allows an external chemical which combines with the external part of the receptor to influence internal cell function without itself entering the cell. 'Chemokines' are cytokines which are concerned with inflammation and attraction of white cells.

10

So is asthma caused by the body not having enough natural beta-2 stimulant on board? Probably not – though it is interesting that certain inherited variants of the gene which carries the code for the beta-2 receptor (on chromosome 5q) affect the severity of disease in asthmatic populations. The body's natural beta-2 stimulant is adrenaline, which (for historical reasons of American patent rights in its name at the time) is known as 'epinephrine' in the USA. This chemical, a 'hormone' (from the Greek verb meaning to arouse or set in motion) can be released into the bloodstream from the adrenal glands, lying above the kidneys at the back of the abdomen. Similar chemicals are released from specialised 'sympathetic' nerves (see p. 32) supplying the airways. One of the reasons why an attack of asthma may get better without drugs is that the combination of panic and lack of oxygen releases adrenaline into the bloodstream. But there is no evidence that lack of adrenaline, or abnormalities in the nerves to the airway muscles, or disorders of the controlling centres in the brain are important causes of asthma.

Steroid drugs

Immediate treatment of a severe asthma attack always involves giving a 'steroid' drug, though the main use of steroids is prophylactic. Prevention of severe or frequent asthma attacks involves regularly inhaling a fine spray of a glucocorticoid steroid drug (e.g. beclomethasone), though long-acting beta-2 stimulants (e.g. salmeterol) are also used to supplement steroids, or to help unusual people who do not respond to steroids. Steroid-resistant asthmatics can also be helped by so-called 'non-steroidal anti-inflammatory drugs' (NSAIDs), for example drugs like indomethacin. This supports the general thesis that asthma is basically an inflammatory condition. Prophylactic drugs, especially steroids, have certainly improved life for asthma sufferers.

What do steroids do? In the airways they reduce 'inflammation'. This term describes the body's reactions to various insults such as bacterial infection, trauma or burns. The features of bacteria-produced inflammation can be seen on the skin as a boil is starting. There is redness, swelling and pain. Under the microscope specialised non-pigmented 'white' blood cells can be seen to leave the bloodstream, accumulate in the inflamed area and destroy invading bacteria. When these cells die and clump together they form pus. People lacking the appropriate white cells resist bacterial infections very badly. Steroids are 'immunosuppressive'. They prevent or diminish allergic inflammatory reactions to inhaled foreign substances.

In such reactions, different white cells from the blood ('eosinophils'

11

and 'mast cells') are commonly found in the lungs. They seem to cause damage by local release of chemicals. Why are normally circulating white blood cells such as eosinophils capable of causing lung damage and inflammatory reactions in asthma? The question has not yet been answered for sure, but a possible explanation is that the normal function of eosinophils is specifically to resist an invasion of the body by small creatures like worms. Worm infestation of the lungs brings forth tremendous quantities of eosinophils which appear to have a normal defensive role. So perhaps eosinophils appear in some cases of asthma because the allergen or whatever is setting off lung inflammation has some similarity to the chemical substances produced by invading animal parasites.

The action of steroids on glucose metabolism means that any substantial excess of steroids in the body can raise the blood sugar and cause diabetes. Fortunately the small amounts of inhaled steroids needed to control asthma do not usually cause trouble. In general, all drugs that specifically interfere with immune and allergic reactions are helpful to asthmatics. A useful prophylactic against asthma, especially in children, is the inhalation of an anti-allergic and IgE-suppressive drug such as chromoglycate. This may allow the dose of steroid drugs to be reduced.

Lung inflammation in asthma

Is there inflammation of the lungs in asthma? There always is. Asthmatics don't get pain in the chest from their lung inflammation, because there are very few pain nerves within the lungs. Redness and swelling of the lungs can't be seen on the skin surface. But when sections of lung are examined under the microscope there is evidence of inflammation around the air passages. We now realise that asthmatics, even when not suffering an attack, have hypersensitive airways which react unduly strongly to irritants or allergens. Such external factors have in common the ability to activate or switch on a large number of genes concerned with inflammation.

The common pathway is an interesting one. Unstimulated cells such as those lining the airways have in their 'cytoplasm' (Greek: 'cyt-' = cell; 'plasm-' = something formed – that part of the cell outside the nucleus) a protein complex called nuclear-factor-kappa-B (NFκB). This is technically a 'transcription factor', which is normally held in an inactive form combined with an inhibitor protein (IκB)[2]. Many forms of stress release NFκB from its inhibitor, thus allowing it to enter the

12

cell nucleus. That is where the transcription takes place. NFκB binds to the controlling elements of DNA and promotes the synthesis of ribose-nucleic acid ('messenger RNA') which is a transcribed copy of the genetic code provided by DNA. This single-stranded nucleic acid molecule then leaves the nucleus and reaches the ribosomes, which manufacture the chemokines involved in lung and airway inflammation. One important effect of steroid drugs – possibly the most important – is to suppress the release of NFκB.

Is asthma triggered by some low-grade chest infection which releases NFκB and switches on production of the damaging inflammatory cytokines? Over the years various candidates have been suggested. A widely distributed bacterium called *Chlamydia pneumoniae* can live inside body cells. When human cells are grown in tissue culture outside the body and then infected with *Chlamydia pneumoniae*, the infected cells produce a variety of cytokines which could be the main cause of lung inflammation in asthma.

Another possibility is that airway inflammation is set off by some non-infective agent. There is recent interest in the particles contained in diesel smoke. Such smoke contains about 100 times more particles per unit volume than petrol engine exhaust gases, even though it is has little immediate constricting effect on airways. Diesel engines now power 25% of road vehicles in the UK. Their use is encouraged on the basis of fuel efficiency, low cost and relatively innocuous gaseous emission; but this takes no account of the production of tiny particles which undoubtedly have the capacity to induce lung inflammation[3].

The cells lining the airways (Fig. 3) are also involved in lung inflam-mation. Most of these cells can release a mixture of cytokines and other chemicals which cause muscle constriction and mucus secretion. There have been several useful summaries of the complex interacting mechanisms[4]. In asthma some of the cells lining the airways are usually swollen. There is also thickening of muscle in the walls of the larger airways. We do not yet know all the ways in which inflamma-tion narrows airways. There may be active muscle constriction, but excessive secretion of mucus is often a more important cause of airway narrowing. There is also increased exudation of fluid directly from the bloodstream. Usually all the airways in an attack of asthma are narrowed by large amounts of thick sticky mucus. The normal ¾ inch (2cm) internal diameter of the trachea may be reduced to little more than a pinhole. Many of the smaller airways become completely plugged with mucus. This is the image of asthma I have in my mind, from the two necropsies I have attended of people who had died in an asthmatic attack.

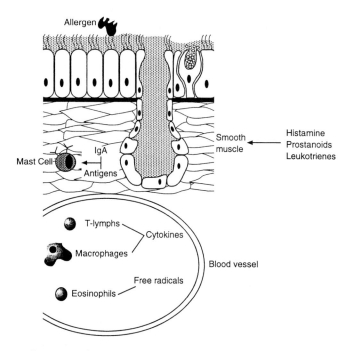

Figure 3 A diagrammatic section through the wall of a small airway (a bronchiole), showing some of the main cells, structures and mechanisms participating in the inflammation and airway narrowing underlying asthma. The cells lining the airway (top of the diagram) contain fine hairs (cilia) which move mucus and foreign particles up the airway towards the mouth, where they are swallowed and removed. In a severe asthma attack the bronchiole would be narrowed by increased mucus secretion and by contraction of the circular 'smooth' muscle cells surrounding the airway.

Effects of airway constriction on gas transport

Asthma can cause death when not enough air is reaching the alveoli of the lungs. Gases can then no longer be exchanged with the blood. Carbon dioxide (CO_2), the waste gas produced during the extraction of energy from food, dissolves readily in the fluid part of blood (the plasma). Any difficulty with excreting carbon dioxide from the lungs can be overcome by the body allowing its concentration (more accurately, its 'partial pressure') to increase. This increases the average gradient for diffusion. People can still stay alive with twice the normal carbon dioxide concentration or even more, though they get a bit drowsy. The big problem with reduced ventilation of the lungs is in oxygen supply. In an attack of asthma many parts of the lungs are

14

blocked off though blood still passes through them. In the alveoli there is a mismatch between ventilation (the movement of air in and out) and perfusion (the passage of blood around the air sacs). It may not be possible to get enough oxygen into the blood to keep the body going. People suffering in a really bad asthma attack need to be artificially ventilated and have the mucus in their airways sucked out.

When people die from asthma the lungs are expanded. Air is sucked in with each deep breath, but can't be breathed out fully because the airways are blocked. It is as if the mucus-filled airways acted as a one-way valve. Failure of lung ventilation may be aggravated by infection (bronchopneumonia) or lung rupture, when air leaks into the space between the lung and the chest wall ('pneumothorax'). I find it difficult to believe that excessive muscular contraction of the airways can by itself cause death, without additional mucus blockage, though some people claim that this is possible. I would expect that such a manifestly disadvantageous situation would have been eliminated by natural selection. If severe mucus blockage is not present in an apparently asthmatic death, it is more likely that there has been a catastrophic heart rhythm disorder rather than obstruction to ventilation.

Leukotriene-receptor antagonists

A recently introduced class of drugs (leukotriene-receptor antagonists, e.g. montelukast and zafirlukast) help to reduce inflammation in asthma by interfering with the ill effects of 'leukotrienes'[5]. These are chemicals released from inflammatory cells and play an important role in airway constriction. Leukotrienes increase the production of sticky mucus and reduce the activity of the 'cilia' (Latin: cilium = eyelid). Cilia are minute hairs lining the airways which beat rhythmically to move particulate matter and mucus up the airways towards the mouth. The effects of leukotriene antagonist drugs add together to make them specially effective. They are a very useful addition or even alternative to steroid drugs.

Hyperventilation in asthma

Although in a bad asthma attack lung ventilation becomes severely obstructed, this does not apply in the early stages of an attack. The amount of air going in and out of the lungs each minute (total ventilation) is often increased, as is the ventilation of the alveoli. This seems paradoxical, but it can happen because lung inflammation itself and low oxygen both send signals to the brain to increase the rate and depth of breathing. It has even been suggested that overbreathing (hyperventilation) is actually the 'cause' of asthma. This is not correct. Many people habitually overbreathe, usually from anxiety, without getting the pathological changes in the lungs which characterise asthma.

But hyperventilation is none the less important. Asthmatics may improve a lot if they are trained to hold their breath and to adopt a slow deliberate breathing pattern. The improvement probably comes because slow breathing gives time for incoming air to warm up. This then reduces the constricting stimulus from cold air. An initial intensive course of steroids to reduce the over-inflation of the lungs will often lead to reduction in hyperventilation and an improvement in symptoms which outlasts the intensive course of steroids. It is always worth making at least one attempt in any severe asthmatic to get rid of every trace of airway narrowing.

Possible environmental factors in the increasing incidence of asthma

So is asthma an allergic reaction to some inhaled material, or is the stage set by the lungs being chronically inflamed or irritated by some constituent of the air we breathe? The answer is probably 'yes' for both possible mechanisms. I have mentioned pollens and the faeces of house-dust mites as potential allergens. British farmers are growing increasing amounts of oil seed rape. Could its pollen be a culprit? A large number of different factors and mediators are undoubtedly involved in causing lung inflammation. These include normal body constituents or products: for example, cytokines, enzymes, transcription factors, prostaglandins, receptor and adhesion molecules, endothelins and nitric oxide. I shall not discuss these any further, even though much therapeutic effort is currently directed towards modifying one or more of these systems. This may eventually provide better control of asthma attacks, but it won't solve the main problem of the increasing incidence of asthma. It is unlikely that people are changing. There must be external factors involved.

Some individuals are allergic to certain foods or chemicals which may trigger off an attack of asthma: for example, peanuts and aspirin. Other environmental contacts (e.g. cats) may also provide allergens. Asthma is getting more common even though the environment in many respects is getting cleaner. Although car exhaust fumes are increasing as the number of cars goes up, no asthma-provoking material in car exhaust emissions has been positively identified, though diesel exhaust fumes are definitely not good for you (see above). Dust particles, crop sprays, refrigeration chemicals and a vast number of other air contaminants are under suspicion. It would be wonderful if we could find the main culprit, if there is a single main one, because then we would have some idea of how to stop asthma getting progressively worse, as it is becoming at present. A huge collaborative epidemiological investigation is under way: the International Study of Asthma and Allergies in Childhood (ISAAC). Self-administered questionnaire data have already been collected on half a million children aged 13–14 in 155 centres in 56 countries[6].

Do animals get asthma? Not often; but domestic cats can get spontaneous asthma attacks. Asthma can be precipitated in cats by exposing them to allergens. This can make their airways narrower, secrete excess amounts of sticky mucus and produce a great increase in eosinophils. Similar reactions to allergens have been produced in human volunteers. However, so far no single allergen has been firmly identified as the main culprit for human asthma, though pollens and house-dust mites certainly make a contribution.

Perhaps there is something in the construction or equipment of modern houses which can trigger asthma in humans and sometimes in cats. Is it that we keep the temperature of modern houses much higher than we used to do, so that some unusual bacterium or virus can flourish? Severe virus infections of the lungs have been observed to predispose to the later development of asthma. Some airborne infections were not identified for many years – for example, so-called 'legionnaires' disease, which is caused by a bacterium which can grow in the hot water tanks of large establishments. (Incidentally, this is why all big hotels now keep their hot water supplies extremely hot, to kill these bacteria).

Is asthma anything to do with television sets? Television tubes need very high voltages (10–20kv) to attract negatively charged electrons to the screen. There is likely to be a cloud of positively charged particles (ions) around the very high voltage transformer, capacitor and screen. Such components electrostatically attract dust, as anyone who has looked at these components inside an old television set knows. Is it possible that clouds of ions around television sets could conceivably accrete and electrically charge dust particles which might act as lung irritants?

There is a tantalisingly large number of other possibilities. It is unlikely that the current increase in asthma incidence can be accounted for by better diagnosis or reporting. Perhaps the reduction of childhood infections, because of better living conditions and increased antibiotic use, increases all allergic responses. This has been suggested as one of the causes for increased asthma incidence. A similar situation has been recognised in other diseases. There is a fascinating animal

17

example. The inbred strain of mice known as 'NOD' spontaneously develop diabetes, probably because of auto-immune destruction of the insulin-secreting cells of their pancreas; but the disease can be completely prevented by infecting young animals with a gut parasite. So it is a plausible hypothesis that asthma may actually be made worse or even precipitated by preventing certain childhood infections.

But this line of reasoning does not explain why domestic cats get asthma. A provocative report has recently come from Ethiopia. In that country asthma is almost unknown in country districts, but common in towns. The particular interest of this report is that diet is hardly different in the two places. There are very few motor vehicles in either place. Atopy in Ethiopia appears to be protective rather than damaging. The authors suggested that the increase in asthma was 'consistent with an effect of new environmental exposures' in towns[7].

Whatever the mysterious environmental factor causing the current nearly worldwide increase in asthma may be, it probably arrives in the air. Some factor or factors peculiar to living in towns seems to be its immediate provocative cause. Apart from my previous suggestion of electrically charged dust particles from television sets, I will make another guess (never previously made by anyone, as far as I am aware) that perhaps polyvinyl chloride (PVC) could be a culprit. PVC is, of course, a solid material. It has never previously been envisaged as a possible cause of the rising non-industrial asthma incidence. But even at room temperature this material in the form of dust is highly irritant and has already been linked to specific asthma risk[8]. Inhalation of PVC smoke by fire-fighters and fire victims can cause prolonged airways hyperresponsiveness, asthma and chronic airways obstruction[9]. Factory work involving PVC processing[10] or meat wrapping or checking[11] can cause respiratory symptoms. PVC is a ubiquitous material in houses. It is used for wrapping food and other goods and for making electrical insulating materials and innumerable other light moulded structures. In the rubbing of coated surfaces which must inevitably accompany normal use, microscopic PVC particles are going to be spread about in the air. Domestic cleaning workers make up one of the occupational groups identified as being specially at risk of asthma[12]. PVC might answer well as a culprit. But the answer will only be given decisively when carefully controlled epidemiological studies have been done. Could PVC be directly damaging, or indirectly damaging through immune sensitisation? Clearly a short exposure to small amounts is harmless but we need to know whether long-continued exposure to PVC dust particles could be a trigger for asthma.

The problem with investigating this or any other possible damaging material lies in determining whether long-lasting exposure over months

18

or years can set up inflammatory processes in the lungs. In the first instance long-range animal studies are needed. It will also be necessary to study matched human population pairs, if enough can be found in which there is a difference in long, continued exposure to some environmental factor such as PVC. This is easier said than done. But such is the nature of all really challenging and important problems.

Summary

'Asthma' describes attacks of difficult breathing due to reversible narrowing of lung airways caused by muscle constriction, swelling of lining cells and secretion of sticky mucus. Force is needed to expel air from the lungs, which become expanded. Gas exchange is impaired. In severe cases lack of oxygen can be fatal.

The disease arises against a background of excessive reaction of lung airways to a variety of external allergic or inflammation-producing agents. Although the immediate precipitating factors are often not known, the final common pathway may involve the release of so-called transcription factors which produce and release inflammation-producing chemicals.

Asthma tends to run in families, but many genes are involved and no simple pattern of inheritance can be found. External factors are probably more important than heredity. The condition is getting commoner, especially in towns, but traffic fumes are probably not its main cause, which has not been identified. Diesel smoke may have slowly developing injurious effects. My own guesses are that charged dust particles around television sets, or minute amounts of PVC (in increasing use in innumerable domestic contexts) might be responsible agents; but hundreds of other possible contenders are under suspicion.

3

MULTIPLE SCLEROSIS

Multiple sclerosis (MS) is the commonest serious neurological disease in many parts of the world. Its incidence in different places varies between 1 and 30 new cases per year for every million population. In the UK about 80,000 people and in the USA about 300,000 have the disease. It characteristically produces episodic and often sudden neurological symptoms and signs. Some of these get better after a few days, but others leave permanent neurological defects. Increasing disability results over the next 30 or 40 years, though the speed of deterioration is extremely variable. Women are two to three times more often affected than men.

Many different neurological functions may be damaged. The commonest damaged parts ('lesions') are the 'upper motor neurone' pathways which control the leg muscles. The word 'neurone'* is used to refer both to the body of a nerve cell and to all the nerve fibres which branch from it. 'Motor' signifies that the neurone is concerned with muscle movements. Upper motor neurones in the outer layers of the brain (the cortex) are linked through nerve fibres with the brain stem and spinal cord (see Fig. 4). A second set of large nerve cells (the 'lower' motor neurones) gives rise to nerve fibres (the anterior nerve roots) directly supplying muscles. The junctions (synapses) between the two sets of nerves allow other neurones to influence the pathway. This makes it possible for a person's conscious intention to make a muscle move (by sending nerve impulses down the motor nerves) to be coordinated by the unconscious automatic harmonised relaxation of opposing muscles and by the contraction of other muscles needed to stabilise joints.

In MS the predominant damage is to upper motor neurones in the brain and spinal cord. Lesions are randomly distributed in nerve tracts, especially in those running close to the central fluid-filled brain cavities (the ventricles). The lesions are usually only the size of a pinhead, but can be larger. Nerve tracts controlling the leg muscles are

---

* The last 'e' is omitted in the USA and many other places, with the expected change in pronunciation.

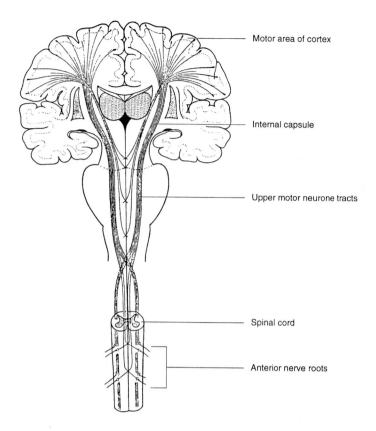

Motor area of cortex

Internal capsule

Upper motor neurone tracts

Spinal cord

Anterior nerve roots

Figure 4 Diagram of the main nerve tracts in the brain and spinal cord which convey electrical impulses to muscles. Multiple sclerosis mainly affects the upper motor neurone tracts. The nerve fibres come from cell bodies in the motor area of the brain cortex and pass down to the brain stem and spinal cord, where they make connection with the lower motor neurones which supply muscles by the anterior nerve roots.

usually interrupted first, probably because they run longer paths. This leads to a stiff ('spastic') weakness of the legs which is the commonest presenting symptom of the disease. Coordination of muscular movement is impaired, often with tremor, because of involvement of the cerebellum (a part of the brain responsible for coordination and balance). Sometimes an episode of double vision lasting a few weeks is the first symptom. This may precede other symptoms by many years.

Different types of MS have been recognised. The commonest (about 80% of cases) occurs in young adults. It is described as 'relapsing/ remitting'. The affected individual runs a stable course between relapses. This form of the disease in about half the cases passes into the 'secondary progressive' form, in which gradual neurological deterioration occurs without discrete sudden relapses. In later life, from the ages of about 40 to 60, the 'primary progressive' form is most common and comprises about 10% of all cases. In this there is a gradual neurological deterioration without any well-marked sudden relapses. Some patients with this form of disease suffer later episodic relapses, in which case the condition is described as 'progressive relapsing'. It is not clear whether these recognisably different manifestations are really different. It may just be a matter of the size of new lesions and the frequency with which they appear.

Sequential studies of the living brain by magnetic resonance imaging (MRI) in all forms of the disease show new lesions regularly appearing and disappearing, though at greatly different rates (see Fig. 5). Those lesions which do not disappear presumably account for

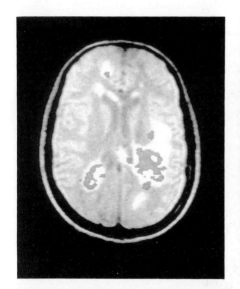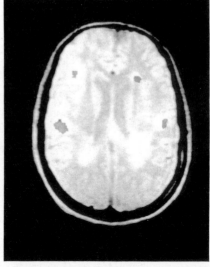

Figure 5 Successive brain MRI scans in a woman of 26 with relapsing/remitting multiple sclerosis which was beginning to enter the secondary progressive phase. The scan on the right was made 3 months after that on the left. The dark blobs (with white surround) on both scans show the site of inflammatory lesions disrupting the blood/brain barrier (identified by a technique involving the injection of a gadolinium compound). Note that all evidence of acute inflammatory foci in the earlier (left hand) scan has disappeared in the later scan, but 4 new small inflammatory lesions have appeared. (Adapted from an original illustration, from McDonald WI and Barnes D, Trends in Neuroscience 1989; 12: 376–379, by permission of Elsevier Science).

persisting neurological defects, though it has proved surprisingly difficult to correlate new MRI-visible lesions with new neurological symptoms.

One reason is that the brain opens up new nerve pathways to bypass damaged neurones. This accounts for the (usually) near-complete recovery of sight in an eye previously blinded by 'retrobulbar neuritis' – a common occurrence in MS. In normal people the main nerve tracts pass from the retina of the eye to an area at the back of the brain, the occipital cortex. After recovery from MS-induced retrobulbar neuritis, dynamic brain imaging reveals that many different connections have been established between the retina and other parts of the brain.

The primary progressive variety of MS is probably the form taken when each successive lesion is so small that the functional defect is difficult for either patient or doctor to recognise when it occurs. Under the microscope, all MS lesions in the brain or spinal cord have in common 'demyelination' of the larger nerve fibres. In the brain and spinal cord these nerve fibres ('axons') are sheathed by an insulating layer of (fat + protein) material called 'myelin'. This allows faster transmission of nerve impulses and insulates each nerve fibre from other adjacent fibres. In MS, in areas which may be only a millimetre or two across, or in much larger patches of disease, the larger nerve fibres lose their normal myelin sheath. The individual lesions of MS seem to arise close to blood vessels, in which there are signs of inflammation and accumulation of blood lymphocytes (see p. 26). Loss of myelin sheaths slows down and impairs nerve impulse transmission, but in many lesions there are also actual axon breaks which make impulse transmission impossible (see below). Fig. 5 shows two successive horizontal MRI scans of the brain in the same patient on two different occasions, 3 months apart. The irregularly shaped dark patches where the blood-brain barrier is disrupted are surrounded by pale areas. Fig. 5 illustrates graphically the dynamic nature of multiple sclerosis, with discrete lesions coming and going.

Genetics

The lifetime risk of developing MS is about 0.2% for the general population in developed countries. There is undoubtedly a genetic element in MS, though an unidentified environmental factor in the home could account for some apparently inherited cases within families. Relatives of patients with MS have a 10–50-fold higher risk of developing the disease than do people without affected relatives. The risk of a brother or sister of an MS patient developing MS is several times increased if the affected individual got the disease early

24

in life. The absolute risk to a first-degree relative (brother, sister, son or daughter of someone with MS) is only about 2–6%. The 'concordance rate' of the disease between twins (the percentage of cases in which a twin is affected when its sibling has the disease) is about 30% for identical ('monozygotic') twins, but only 2% for non-identical ('dizygotic') twins. Genetic influence must involve several gene differences. An external environmental factor or factors is evidently much more important than heredity.

Epidemiology

The disease is commoner in cold northern climates than in hot countries. It is commoner in cool southern parts in the Southern hemisphere than in the warm northern parts (e.g. of Australia). This is not a universal rule; it does not, for example, apply to Japan. Within Europe the distribution of cases does not bear out any clear relation to geographical latitude, but the enormous differences in incidence in different places in the world certainly point towards an environmental factor. Ultraviolet light appears to be immunosuppressive. It has been suggested that sunlight may protect against MS because of this, and account for some of the geographical differences in incidence.

Cause

Studies of people migrating to different environmental areas at different periods of life suggest that whatever the environmental factor may be, it is acquired before puberty[1]. Adolescence seems to be a critical time for later developing MS. The different attack rate in different geographical areas may give us clues about the possible cause of the disease. A virus[*] infection seems much the most probable environmental trigger. The anti-viral agent beta-interferon can reduce relapse rate and may perhaps modify the course of the disease, though many questions remain.

Many viruses are known selectively to attack specific parts of the brain and spinal cord. 'Polio' is a good example. The poliomyelitis virus has been firmly established as the cause of that disease. The damaged parts of the brain can be identified under the microscope and

---

[*] Whereas bacteria are minute single-celled living organisms, viruses are smaller and can be thought of as inanimate packets of nucleic acid and other chemicals, which on entry to a body cell can stimulate it to produce more of its own material.

virtually complete protection can be provided by immunisation with a preparation derived from inactivated virus.

Though there have been reports of clusters of cases of MS in some restricted locations (e.g. in the Hebrides), it is exceedingly difficult to establish whether these are outside the bounds of statistical chance. Also, in defined regions in which the disease has been well-studied the annual incidence of newly-diagnosed cases is very variable over time. This is characteristic of most epidemics of infectious disease. There has been some evidence suggesting that bird viruses might be involved[2]. A promising lead suggests that a recently discovered retrovirus[*] is strongly associated with MS and is only rarely found in normal individuals[3]. It has also been suggested that infection with Epstein-Barr(E-B) virus (technically a ubiquitous 'B-lymphotropic' herpes virus which causes glandular fever when acquired in adult life) may pave the way for a retrovirus infection which triggers MS in susceptible individuals. Another virus which can attack the nervous system is Japanese encephalitis virus (JEV), which can be acquired from pigs and spread by mosquitoes. In parts of South-East Asia many children are infected, with little morbidity, but infection acquired later in life can give rise to neuronal damage resembling poliomyelitis. This scenario resembles infection with the E-B virus: childhood infection often harmless but infection acquired as an adult potentially damaging.

Progressive multifocal leucoencephalopathy (PML) is an interesting virus infection which produces ill effects more or less exclusively in so-called 'immunocompromised' patients whose immune defences are seriously impaired. This commonly occurs in infections by the human immunodeficiency virus (HIV), which causes 'acquired immunodeficiency syndrome' (commonly abbreviated to AIDS). PML is almost unknown in normal individuals, but has occurred in as many as 5% of AIDS patients, whose specialised protective 'T'-lymphocytes[+] in the blood are severely reduced in numbers. PML is due to infection with a usually harmless papovavirus, known as the 'JC' virus (so named from

[*] a name given to a virus which gets into a cell by the back door, so to speak. It uses a facilitating protein (an enzyme) called 'reverse transcriptase' to insert its own genetic code into the genetic code of the host cell. This then instructs the cell's ribosomes to make more copies of the virus, thus perpetuating the infection.

[+] The 'T-'lymphocytes make up a substantial proportion of the 'white' cells of the blood – those not containing the red pigment haemoglobin. After appropriate priming they directly attack foreign cells or foreign material. The 'B-' lymphocytes exert their protective function indirectly by producing soluble proteins ('antibodies') which combine with and inactivate potentially damaging chemicals or cells. Their protective action is thus exerted at a distance, whereas 'T'-lymphocytes are themselves intimately involved in protective immune reactions.

the first patient in whom it was recognised). Since antibodies to JC virus can be detected in more than 70% of normal adults, infection is obviously harmless to most people. The situation is similar to that of E-B virus, mentioned above. Since PML can produce clinical symptoms and brain image changes looking very much like MS on X-rays and MRI scans, the virus has been looked for in MS. However, neither this nor any other virus, apart perhaps from the recently reported retrovirus, has so far been convincingly identified and confirmed in the brain cells of MS patients. Though the evidence is not strong enough to incriminate any specific virus at present, a virus trigger for MS seems still the most likely primary cause of the disease.

Immunological aspects

There are many reasons to suppose that the body's immune defence system is in some way involved in causing or perpetuating the disease[4]. There is a statistically-verified association of MS with the 'human leucocyte antigen'[*] (HLA) system[5]. In addition there are two recognised influences on relapse rate in those already diagnosed with MS. In the period from two weeks before until five weeks after the onset of one of the common virus infections, the relapse rate of MS increases nearly threefold. Although pregnancy does not alter the natural history of the disease, relapse frequency is much reduced during the last three months of pregnancy, but much increased in the three months after delivery. Virus infections are believed to activate the body's immune system. Specific changes in anti-inflammatory T-lymphocytes occur towards the end of pregnancy and reverse after delivery. Sudden deterioration, usually coinciding with the appearance of a new MRI-identifiable lesion in the brain, can usually be reversed

[*] An 'antigen' (Greek 'anti-' = against; 'gen' = to produce) is a chemical compound or part of an organism which can induce an immune reaction when it enters or comes into contact with appropriate receptors. The presentation and occurrence of components of the human leucocyte (white cell) antigen (HLA) system are genetically controlled. Antigens already in the body before birth are described as 'auto-antigens'. Unless changes occur in disease they are accepted as part of 'self' and do not excite immune reactions. The well-known chemicals determining the blood groups A and B are examples of antigens which can cause transfusion reactions in people who have antibodies against them. (I used to be puzzled to know why Group A people had antibodies to the Group B antigen, and vice versa. I thought that this was because blood group antigens are present in saliva and that the universal practice of kissing new-born babies exposed them to a wide variety of antigens. But I later found that the main blood group chemicals are ubiquitous enough to make this mechanism superfluous!)

27

or cut short by giving large doses of steroids (immunosuppressive glucocorticoid drugs such as prednisone and methylprednisone).

Conditions closely similar to MS can be produced in animals by repeated exposure to certain provocative agents, including components of myelin, the (fat + protein)-containing material ensheathing large nerve fibres. The suggestion has often been made that there is a vicious circle in MS. Destruction of myelin might lead to exposure of the body's immune system to myelin components. These might then produce further immune reactions directed towards myelin, whose destruction might then complete a vicious circle. It seems possible that a vicious circle of this sort might be started by a virus infection and later be kept going by the body's own immunological system, without the original virus necessarily being involved[5]. But if so why should the disease affect different parts of the nervous system at different times?

Demyelination and axon breaks

Hitherto a lot of research has concentrated on finding the cause of demyelination. People have tried to control MS by supplying extra dietary amounts of some of the chemical constituents of myelin. The oil of the evening primrose is a popular though unproven remedy. However, careful microscopic examination of axons (the central threadlike structures conducting nerve impulses) in MS lesions has revealed that there are actual breaks in many axons, with egg-shaped swellings at the breaks. Such observations were made more than a century ago by the French neurologist Jean Charcot. They have been recently intensively studied[6]. They rather convincingly explain why permanent neurological impairment can follow a sudden worsening of neurological symptoms, although the possibility has to be considered that loss of myelin sheaths comes first and makes axons unduly fragile.

Therapeutic efforts need to be directed towards prevention of MS rather than cure since reversal of established lesions seems hopelessly optimistic. Some protection against attacks of brain inflammation, easily identified by MRI, has been achieved by the selective removal of specialised T-lymphocytes by injecting an appropriate antibody. The idea is that such lymphocytes are immunologically active cells which are destroying myelin. The long term merit of this treatment is uncertain, especially as it may cause auto-immune disease of the thyroid gland.

Summary

MS is a common disabling neurological disease. It may start in early adult life, with an episode of double vision or difficulty in walking.

Progression is usually via brief attacks in which symptoms increase and disabilities develop. Some attacks clear up completely, but others result in permanent loss of function.

The condition is probably initiated by infection with a virus, which may be an as yet unknown retrovirus. The infection is probably acquired in childhood or adolescence. It is commoner in colder parts of the world than hotter. This might mean that transmission of the virus from person to person is commoner where people live closely together in poorly-ventilated rooms with the windows shut and rarer in hotter places where there is less overcrowding and windows stay open. Such ideas suggest that infection may be acquired by breathing in the exhalations of infected people. The initial infection may lead to a state in which neurological damage progresses because of damaging reactions by the body's immunological protection systems. This self-sustaining condition might not necessarily involve further virus replication.

Other routes of infection are possible. I don't know the figures, but would suspect that infestation of houses by rodents is commoner in temperate climates, so that chance contact of humans with rodents is greater. Rats in particular are known to carry many diseases which infect man. There is no convincing epidemiological evidence incriminating domestic animals of any sort. Perhaps we need some 'lateral thinking' to identify other possible routes for a virus infection, for example, through diet. Hepatitis A is a virus infection of the liver usually acquired through eating or drinking material contaminated with the virus.

Complete solution of the mystery of MS will not necessarily lead to an immediate cure or 100% prevention. AIDS is an example of a virus infection where understanding of the cause of the disease has come long before its cure has been established. However, seeing the rapid progress now being made in slowing down or arresting progression of HIV infection, I am hopeful that once the causative agent or agents of MS has been identified, control or suppression of the disease will soon follow. I expect that this will come about within the next decade.

4

FAINTING

The Greek word 'syncope' (pronounced 'sin-co-pee') strictly means a 'cutting short' or a swoon, i.e. a sudden loss of consciousness. A faint is a particular kind of syncope. Physicians often describe a faint as 'vaso-vagal' or 'neurocardiogenic' syncope, for reasons which will be explained later.

The most dramatic faint that I have ever seen took place at an international conference in which a distinguished scientist was about to deliver a lecture on – ironically – the physiology of veins. He had been seated listening to an appropriately flattering introduction. He stood up, said 'Mr Chairman, ladies and gentlemen...' when his voice faded, he passed out and fell to the ground. Although he quickly regained consciousness, he had to abandon his lecture. I took him out to lunch and gave him a lot of salty soup, though in fact he had already fully recovered. He was unlucky. It was a high prestige occasion; he was nervous; the hall was hot; he had been sitting down for some time before.

What is the mystery? Surely someone faints when the blood pressure gets too low and not enough blood is going to the brain. Correct! But it's not quite that simple. The first thing to note is that people who are lying down flat don't faint. Indeed it is exceptionally rare even for anyone sitting in a chair to faint. The victim of a faint has to be standing. Someone who is slowly bleeding to death on the ground will just as slowly lose consciousness as his blood pressure slowly falls. In a faint, on the other hand, a lot of things happen very suddenly. The blood pressure falls sharply in the space of a few seconds. Consciousness is lost. A victim who is standing falls to the ground.

Normal control of the circulation during standing

So let me start by describing the things that normally happen when someone stands up. Gravity drags some of the circulating blood towards the feet. Elastic blood vessels expand a bit and allow some blood to pool in the lower parts of the body. This reduces the effective volume of circulating blood. The heart can't pump so much blood round. The blood pressure therefore starts to fall. But within a few seconds it comes back to normal because:

1 The fall of blood pressure is detected by pressure sensors in the main arteries and in the heart chambers. These connect to the brain via nerves.
2 The brain coordinates the information and sends messages down nerves connected to contractile blood vessels, especially those in the lower parts of the body (the leg veins in particular). This makes them contract and squeeze blood towards the heart. The heart therefore fills up better.
3 The brain also sends messages in nerves to the heart, making it speed up and contract more vigorously.

The 'autonomic' nervous system

All these reactions are brought about by the autonomic[*] nervous system whose control centres are in the brain stem, right at the back and base of the skull. The control centres get second-by-second information about the blood pressure not only in the large neck arteries but also in the veins from which blood flows to fill the heart. This information is transmitted by specialised nerve endings in the walls of these vessels and in the walls of the heart itself. Although these specialised nerve endings detect stretch, in effect they sample blood pressure. Hence they are known as 'baroreceptors' (Greek: baro- = pressure). The information is transmitted in the form of bursts of electrical impulses, conveyed by the 'vagus' nerves running up each side of the neck. The rate of discharge of nerve impulses increases when the pressure (and hence the stretch of the vessel wall) is increased.

The control centres in the brain stem are getting all this information continuously, every second of our lives, day and night. The brain automatically brings about appropriate corrective action. It is a classic negative feedback system. If the blood pressure falls for any reason (e.g. standing up or losing blood), the brain corrects the fall. Specialised 'sympathetic' nerves (part of the autonomic nervous system) go

---

[*] 'Autonomic' implies that this part of the central nervous system is automatic and virtually outside the control of the will. Most of the control centres are in the brain stem and midbrain, though higher brain centres also connect with the brain stem. The two main components of the system are the 'sympathetic' (mainly constricting blood vessels and increasing the heart rate and force of contraction) and the 'parasympathetic' (slowing down the heart rate via the vagus nerves and dilating some blood vessels). The reader who has not encountered these terms needs to understand that 'sympathetic' in this context is a purely technical term: there is no other name for this system of nerves. It has no emotional significance!

from the brain stem to the veins and arteries, making them constrict so that the blood in the circulation is gripped more tightly. Other sympathetic nerves increase the force and rate of contraction of the heart. Consequently the blood pressure is brought back to its normal level.

What happens during a faint?

During a faint something goes wrong. A recent (1996) reviewer commented: 'The cardiovascular system is striving to maintain an adequate blood pressure. What suddenly switches off this compensation ... remains one of the most intriguing mysteries in cardiovascular physiology'[1]. Instead of the heart gradually beating faster it suddenly slows right down. Instead of the veins and arteries continuing to contract they suddenly dilate. Consequently blood pressure falls sharply. The flow of blood to the brain becomes inadequate. The victim loses consciousness and falls to the ground. The faint is preceded by the skin becoming pale and sweaty. There is often accompanying nausea.

The sequence of events has been carefully studied by experiments on normal volunteers on tilt tables. Fig. 6 shows on a realistic timescale a diagram of the circulatory changes in a normal young man tilted head-up in warm room. For the first few minutes (from A to B) blood pressure was falling slightly, heart rate was gradually increasing and muscle blood flow in arms and legs was decreasing. The blood pressure was being maintained by increased activation of the sympathetic nervous system. This corrected the effects of gravity by increasing resistance to blood flow in the arteries (so-called 'peripheral resistance'), by constricting veins, and by increasing the heart rate. At point B the subject complained of nausea and his skin became pale and sweaty. Then all of a sudden the peripheral resistance fell. Arteries previously constricted suddenly dilated. The heart slowed right down (point C in Fig. 6). The blood in the arteries was no longer at a high enough pressure to supply the brain with enough blood. Our subject fainted. Fortunately the whole system started to reverse as soon as he lay flat (point D). The heart speeded up again. Arteries and veins constricted again. Within seconds everything was back to normal (point E).

Such events have often been witnessed by thousands watching military parades in hot weather. It is commonplace for an entirely fit young male soldier, standing stock still, to lose consciousness and fall to the ground as if poleaxed.

The activities of the autonomic nervous system, especially of its

33

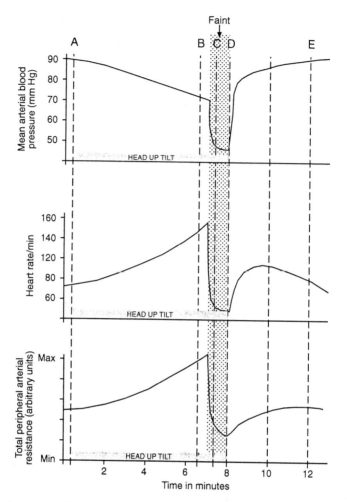

Figure 6 Sequence of events in the minutes before, during and after a faint, induced in a normal supine adult volunteer by head up tilting in a warm room. The appropriate compensatory mechanisms were maintaining blood pressure and adequate brain blood supply until the blood pressure fell suddenly and the subject lost consciousness (see text).

sympathetic division, have been studied during fainting by directly recording nerve impulses from an accessible sympathetic nerve, usually in the leg. This can be done by pushing ultra-thin needles (insulated except at the tip) through the skin and into a nerve trunk. Such records show that until the moment of the faint the rate of discharge of electrical impulses in sympathetic nerves going to arteries supplying the leg muscles progressively increases. This makes the arteries constict. But at the moment of a faint everything reverses. The rate of discharge of impulses in sympathetic nerves gets less and may stop altogether. Blood pressure drops sharply and the heart rate slows. The force of contraction of heart muscle also diminishes. The changes in heart function are mostly brought about by increased nervous discharge in the vagus nerves, which run from the hind brain to the heart. These 'parasympathetic' nerves are also part of the autonomic nervous system, but they have mainly opposite effects to those of the sympathetic nerves. It is possible to remove the cardiac component of fainting by injecting the drug atropine, commonly known as 'belladonna' (beautiful lady: so called because it makes the pupils dilate). After giving atropine and tilting someone upright, the heart rate does not slow down. Despite this subjects can still be made to faint.

Fainting has been induced and studied in human volunteers by various combinations of head-up tilt, blood pressure lowering drugs, blood loss, blood pooling with leg cuffs, lower body negative pressure and emotional trauma. It may be aggravated by heat, fever, coughing, passing urine or lack of oxygen. The results have been strikingly consistent and conform exactly to the sequence of events shown in Fig. 6. The faint itself is accompanied by sweating and by massive secretion of various powerful circulating chemicals (hormones). But however severe it may be, a faint can always be terminated at once by putting the subject flat, or head down, when all the changes reverse within seconds.

Cause

'There is no more dramatic or thoroughly investigated cardiovascular response than the everyday common faint'[2]. The current and now conventional view of its cause was first propounded in 1972. It was suggested that fainting is caused by 'increased activity of the [nerve] receptors located in the left ventricle [of the heart] ... with rapid bleeding or pooling of blood, the receptors are excited by an improper squeezing of the myocardium when the ventricles contract vigorously around an almost empty chamber ... it seems reasonable to conclude that they [ventricular receptors] are, to a large extent, responsible for triggering this response'[3]. I think that this explanation is wrong, or at best incomplete.

Here is a more recent verdict: 'A link between ventricular receptor activity and the vasovagal reaction [i.e. the faint] is not firmly established. It has not even been demonstrated that there is a net increase in ventricular [baroreceptor nervous] activity after hemorrhage'[4]. Karl

35

Popper has pointed out that although no amount of supportive evidence ever proves a case, a scientific hypothesis may be refuted by a single piece of contradictory evidence. Such evidence is now available. Typical faints have been observed in cardiac transplant patients. Such patients have had both ventricles replaced and all ventricular nerves cut. In one patient studied, after infusion of a drug which dilated blood vessels, 'classic vasovagal symptoms suddenly developed ... accompanied by the abrupt cessation of sympathetic discharge. From these observations, we conclude that vasodilator-induced syncope is not always dependent on ventricular baroreceptor activation'[5]. Although heart transplantation removes the cardiac ventricles it leaves behind the posterior walls of the two atria. Many sensory nerve endings in the atria and great veins will inevitably survive. Fig. 7 shows the normal human heart viewed from the front. The right and left ventricles (horizontal line-shading) are sacrificed before transplantation. The remaining back walls of the two atria and the superior vena cava (dotted shading) are left. It is notable that after cardiac transplantation 'Afferents from the remnant atria, venoarterial junctions, pulmonary veins ... are left intact'[5]. Why could not vasovagal syncope be triggered from these receptors rather than from the ventricles?

Fainting can, as I have suggested elsewhere[6], be best accounted for by the sudden collapse of unfilled atria (especially the right atrium) and of unfilled great veins. This could send misleading information to the brain, telling it that the heart was over- rather than under-filled. Consequent dilation of arteries and veins would decrease right atrial pressure still further and lead to a vicious circle (Fig. 8). This would explain the abrupt nature of the faint. Many years ago I was recording from nerves in the neck of anaesthetised cats. These were conveying electrical impulses from the heart to the brain. I noticed that there were numerous nerves coming from receptors in the atria and great veins but relatively few from receptors located in the cardiac ventricles. It was easy to increase the rate of discharge of nerve impulses by lightly pressing the front wall of the right atrium. Inward collapse of the atrial wall would therefore be expected to lead to increased nerve impulse discharge rate of atrial stretch receptors. Even in the more rigid carotid artery it has been observed that when internal pressure falls to zero, or close to it, the discharge rate of the baroreceptors in the carotid sinus wall paradoxically increases. This phenomenon is known as 'collapse firing' of these receptors.

This explanation for fainting is supported by a brief report[7] that when nerve impulses coming from atrial stretch receptors were recorded during experimental haemorrhage the discharge rate notably

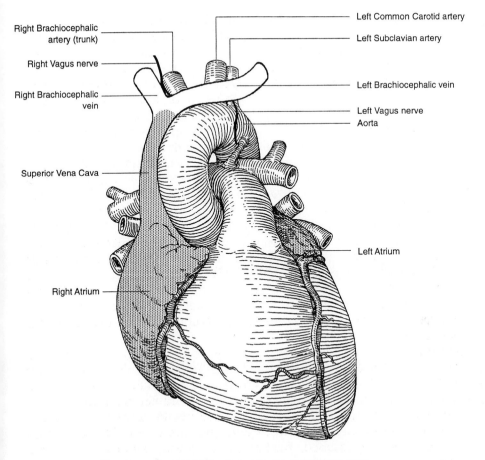

Right Brachiocephalic artery (trunk)

Right Vagus nerve

Right Brachiocephalic vein

Superior Vena Cava

Right Atrium

Left Common Carotid artery

Left Subclavian artery

Left Brachiocephalic vein

Left Vagus nerve
Aorta

Left Atrium

Shaded areas show distribution of low pressure baro/stretch receptors

Figure 7 Diagram of the heart and main blood vessels seen from the front. Horizontal line shading shows the two ventricles, with coronary arteries on their surface. The fine shaded areas – the right atrium, superior vena cava and left atrium – have in their walls the low pressure stretch receptors (venous baroreceptors). These send nerve impulses up to the brain via the vagus nerves on each side.

increased. My emphasis on the low-pressure side of the systemic circulation is also compatible with old observations by the late E.P.Sharpey-Schafer, who made many of the seminal clinical studies of fainting. He noted that congestive heart failure in man, in which the circulation is overfilled and pressure in the right atrium and great veins is greatly increased, gave 'immunity from vaso-vagal syncope' – exactly as my hypothesis would predict.

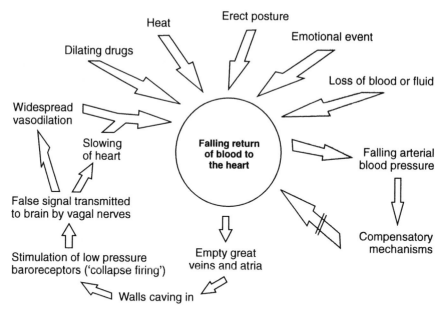

Figure 8 Hypothetical but plausible vicious circle, showing precipitating factors leading to falling blood pressure and to a sequence of events which – if compensatory mechanisms are not powerful enough – could cause slowing of the heart and widespread dilation of blood vessels, leading to fainting.

There is considerable, though not unanimous, evidence which I have reviewed elsewhere[6] that increased nerve impulse traffic from atrial stretch receptors causes reflex dilation of blood vessels and slowing of the heart. So far, so good. But the effects of atrial distension on heart rate are less clear-cut. Increased pressure in the right side of the heart in dogs and cats has been recorded as causing slowing of the heart, through a vagus nerve-mediated reflex. But in other circumstances opposite effects on heart rate have been observed. However, all the available evidence suggests that the normal physiological response to increased discharge from atrial and atrio-venous baroreceptors is dilation of systemic arteries and veins. This is exactly what happens at the start of a faint. There is no reliable evidence to contradict my premise that the normal physiological response to increased venous baroreceptor discharge, at least at high initial heart rates, is slowing of the heart. This is the other component of the vaso-vagal response.

Though the evidence in favour of my hypothesis is strong, it is not of course conclusive. Indeed, as a follower of Karl Popper, I must accept that there is no such thing as a scientific proof of anything. We have to work at all times on the balance of probabilities given the evidence available at the time. I have tried, so far without success, to persuade someone with the necessary facilities to join me in looking via ultrasound imaging of human subjects, at the cavity of the right atrium as the faint begins, to see whether it collapses inwards precisely at that moment, as I predict. I also predict that it should be possible for a subject to initiate a faint prematurely by trying to breathe out against resistance (e.g. by blowing up a balloon). This should make the low pressure atria and large veins in the chest collapse.

Fortunately these are such simple experiments that I am hopeful that a definitive answer will soon be forthcoming. In the meantime, the current opinion of most physiologists is that the cardiac ventricles are primarily involved, and/or that the faint reaction is coordinated in the brain. I am suggesting, in this heretical chapter, that the cardiac ventricles play no important part in initiating fainting and that the brain is getting its misleading information from low pressure receptors in atria and large veins. But whether I am right or wrong, I hope the reader will agree that fainting is one of the most fascinating medical mysteries around.

Summary

Fainting is a strange reaction which can occur in people standing upright who remain very still, lose blood or in some other way suffer a gradual fall of blood pressure. Suddenly the heart rate (which had been hitherto increasing) slows right down. Systemic arteries (which had been progressively constricting) open up. The blood pressure falls dramatically, within a few seconds. There is then not enough blood going to the brain and the individual faints. Before the faint 'the cardiovascular system is striving to maintain an adequate blood pressure. What suddenly switches off this compensation ... remains one of the most intriguing mysteries in cardiovascular physiology'[1].

I have suggested[6] that 'collapse firing' of low-pressure baro(stretch)-receptors in the right atrium and great veins, and possibly on the left side of the heart as well, is a plausible and sufficient explanation for the sequence of events in fainting. The central effects of such inappropriate information coming to the brain are dilation of systemic blood vessels and slowing of the heart. Activation of ventricular muscle receptors is neither a probable nor a necessary cause of fainting, though it might play an additional part in the response. This hypothesis explains logically why fainting does not occur in the presence of congestive heart failure and why it can still be observed in patients who have had heart transplants.

If at the moment the faint occurs the right atrium and/or great veins do not suddenly collapse inwards the hypothesis is disproved. The atria and great veins can easily be watched moment to moment via ultrasound imaging, which can show the outline of these low-pressure vessels without even puncturing the skin. The court awaits the verdict.

5

PSORIASIS

Psoriasis is a common inflammatory skin condition which at some time in their lives affects 1–3% of the world's population, more than 2% of Europeans and about 8 million people in the USA. It typically produces sharply demarcated scaly raised red plaques or patches. The lesions are usually roughly symmetrical. The elbows, knees, back of the forearm and back of the upper arm are commonly involved, as well as the scalp, penis and vulva (Fig. 9). These are all places where there is pressure or rubbing, both of which seem to be provocative factors. But in severe cases almost the whole skin surface can be involved. The nails are often pitted and deformed, especially if the disease has also involved the joints (psoriatic arthropathy). The joint disease produces deformities, especially of the hands, which resemble rheumatoid arthritis (see Chapter 8), though the rheumatoid factor (see p. 72) in psoriatic arthropathy is negative.

In Dennis Potter's BBC television play *The Singing Detective* the chief character spent a long period in hospital being treated for extensive psoriasis with joint involvement. The realistic depiction of his sufferings came from the author's own experiences. He was able to dramatise his illness in this unusual vicarious manner. The American novelist John Updike has also dramatised the sufferings of the severely affected psoriatic from his personal knowledge. For most people psoriasis is fortunately a mild, though tiresome, disease. It affects general health very little unless large areas of skin are involved, or if there is much inflammation, as there can be in generalised pustular psoriasis.

Psoriasis can appear at any age but it typically appears for the first time between 20 and 25, though there is another smaller peak around age 50. It does not shorten life. Although there is excessive growth and proliferation of certain skin layers, psoriasis does not itself predispose to cancer, although certain treatments make use of controlled exposure to ultraviolet light, which can cause skin cancer. Some people have even suggested that cancer may be less common in people with psoriasis than in those without the condition. Long term controlled epidemiological studies are needed. There seems to be a relative excess

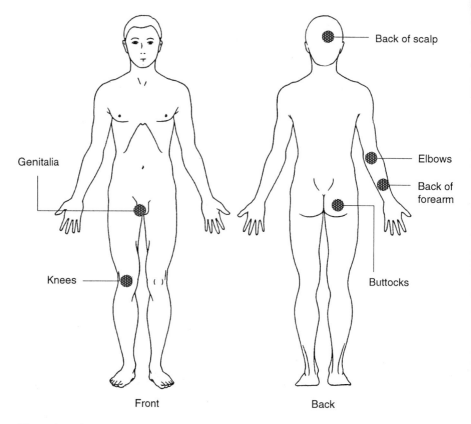

Genitalia

Knees

Front

Back of scalp

Elbows

Back of forearm

Buttocks

Back

Figure 9 Diagrams showing the common sites of psoriatic lesions.

of factors encouraging growth of blood vessels and of the outer layer of the skin (the 'epidermis', from Greek 'epi' = upon/above; 'dermis' = skin). There is also a relative deficiency of factors normally suppressing growth of blood vessels. (Blood vessel growth and prevention of growth are discussed further in Chapter 21).

A number of other skin conditions look like psoriasis in their early stages, but the outstanding characteristic is the absence or relative mildness of itching, compared with conditions such as seborrhoeic dermatitis, chronic eczema and drug-induced eruptions, in which itching is usually more severe. (It is ironic that the word 'psoriasis' derives from Greek: 'psora' = itch.) The other clue is a positive family history. This is commonly found, especially in people whose psoriasis started early in life. In case of doubt a biopsy (Greek: 'bios' = life; 'opsis' = sight) of a skin lesion is examined under the light microscope. On the surface of affected skin there is a thick layer of scale, a hard insoluble protein-containing crust, with loss of the layer of cells just beneath it. (The word 'keratin' – Greek: 'keras' = horn – has a less specific meaning, and 'scale' is the preferred term.)

There is also excessive growth and enlargement of blood vessels in the deeper layers of the skin. The epidermis is abnormally thickened, even in areas where the skin appears normal to the naked eye. The rich network of blood vessels in psoriatic lesions can be shown by gently scraping their scaly surface. This (painless) procedure produces minute drops of blood on the surface of the lesions.

Cause

In the affected parts of the skin there appears to be a great (tenfold) increase in the rate of growth of the cells which form the epidermal layer. Apparently normal skin also shows an increase in cell growth rate, though the turnover rate of cells is not as rapid as in the lesions themselves. It is difficult to measure skin cell turnover rate and to grow scale-forming cells in tissue culture; but estimates of replication rate suggest that the rate can probably vary from one cell division per day to one every month. Scales presumably form when the rate of growth of the epidermis exceeds the rate of cell destruction. An underlying defect in psoriasis seems to be in the processes concerned with wound healing.

When fibre-forming cells in skin from psoriatic patients are grown in tissue culture, completely outside the body, it has been reported (though not yet confirmed) that they synthesise at a faster rate than normal a fibre protein called 'collagen', which is important in skin structure. We don't know whether the problem is excessive stimulation of the cell division cycle, or whether there is reduced activity of inhibitors of cell growth. Curiously, despite the increased growth rate, skin thickness is not increased in uninvolved skin in psoriasis.

Many possible causal factors have been studied, but no single one has been incriminated as the main functional defect in psoriasis. Increased production of inflammation-promoting factors such as IL-1β, IL-6 and TNFα, and IL-8[*] is particularly notable, but the reason for the excessive production of these cytokines is not known. Recent discoveries in asthma have revealed the key role of NFκB in switching on the transcription of genes coding for inflammation-mediating cytokines (see p.

---

[*] 'IL' is the abbreviation of 'interleukin' and TNF of 'tumour necrosis factor': all these are 'cytokines'.

12). I anticipate that NFκB in scale-forming skin cells is likely to play a key role in the inflammation which characterises psoriasis. There has already been a hint of this possibility[1].

The importance of genes is shown by the frequent occurrence of a family history, especially in those who develop severe symptoms early in life. After the initial report of a gene locus on chromosome 17, which is now recognised as specially linked to psoriatic arthropathy, other genes on chromosomes 2, 8 and 20 have been weakly linked with psoriasis. A gene or genes on chromosome 6 (at 6p21) is the strongest genetic link so far identified[2]. The inheritance is evidently polygenic. What is inherited seems to be a predisposition which needs an environmental stimulus for its expression, as in so many of the medical mysteries described in this book. Studies of identical twins have shown that both twins do not necessarily develop psoriasis even if one has it[3], though concordance rates are high. Environmental factors may be as important as genes.

Immunological factors

The fact that steroid drugs (glucocorticoids) can reduce inflammation in psoriasis is compatible with an auto-immune cause. It does not prove the causal association because steroids suppress the production of many inflammation-producing cytokines. Stopping steroids can exacerbate the disease. But on the other hand complete disappearance of psoriatic lesions can only rarely be obtained by the use of steroids, which in any case sometimes seem to destabilise scaly skin and make it pustular.

Psoriasis is reported to have been transmitted to a previously normal individual by a bone marrow transplant from a patient with psoriasis. This probably means that T-lymphocytes themselves can initiate the disease. The involvement of these cells in causing psoriatic lesions is also supported by ingenious (though as yet unconfirmed) animal experiments in which mice were made immunodeficient so that they could tolerate a graft of human skin. Then it was found that lymphocytes from patients with psoriasis, even when taken from apparently normal skin, could induce the changes of psoriasis in human skin grafts in the mice[4].

There is an association of psoriasis with certain specific inherited human leucocyte antigens (HLA: see p. 27), especially Cw6 and DR7. The association with HLA Cw6 is particularly close in young people. None the less, only 10% of people with this antigen develop the disease. The type of disease described as generalised pustular psoriasis has a different genetic HLA association, with A1, B37 and DRw10.

Although particular HLA antigens may confer susceptibility to psoriasis, they are not of great causal significance. The inheritance of psoriasis, like most conditions of variable severity, certainly involves many genes. Probably a genetic predisposition from the HLA system needs to coincide with one, or a few, additional common genetic variations.

These associations suggest that psoriasis may be an 'auto-immune T-cell disease' (see p. 26). Much collateral evidence suggests that a predisposition to develop auto-immunity is an inherited 'dominant trait' (see p. 60) and that HLA genes determine the type of auto-immunity. The effectiveness of immunosuppressive drugs such as cyclosporine and azathioprine is a further pointer towards psoriasis involving a T-cell auto-immune response.

Although experiments in animals have not yet brought a break-through to solve the enigma of psoriasis, the creation of 'transgenic' mice has opened up an enormous field of research in which the human genes determining the severity, type and location of psoriatic lesions will be gradually identified. Although psoriasis is not unique to man and has been observed in primates, typical lesions have not been identified in lower animals, though mice can develop a large variety of scaly skin conditions.

Environmental triggers

Environmental factors may be nearly as important as heredity. Obesity, smoking and certain drugs aggravate psoriasis. Lithium (a treatment for serious depressive illness) has been recorded as making psoriatic lesions worse. The importance of psychological factors is disputed, though physical or emotional stress sometimes appear to be trigger factors. I remember a striking case. On the first day a colleague was to start a particularly responsible and demanding medical job he had to be admitted to hospital for a bad attack of psoriasis affecting his entire body.

However, it is unwise to make deductions from anecdotes surrounding such a common disease. Physical trauma (the Koebner effect) is probably an aggravating factor, accounting for the localisation of psoriatic plaques on areas such as the elbows which are often pressed and rubbed. Mechanical strain may release the powerful cytokine (see p. 10) IL-1α, which promotes the inflammatory reaction.

Infection and psoriasis

The appearance of new lesions has often seemed to follow a strepto-coccal sore throat, suggesting that the *Streptococcus haemolyticus* bacterium is a cause of psoriasis. Anti-streptococcal antibiotics may improve the disease. Streptococci have been found in the skin lesions of a few patients who have responded well to antibiotics. There are close chemical similarities between some of the proteins from streptococcal bacteria and keratin protein in normal human skin. So perhaps the body starts treating its own skin scale as if it was an invading bacterial organism. There is also an association between psoriasis and infections with the bacterium *Staphylococcus aureus*, which causes boils and other skin infections.

Streptococcal and staphylococcal bacteria can both embody 'superantigens', a group of proteins which can activate many different T-cells[5]. Some people have suggested that psoriasis is a T-cell mediated auto-immune reaction (see p.26) triggered by bacterial superantigens, releasing damaging cytokines. So far the jury is out. These 'pyogenic' (pus-producing) infections may not be essential to maintain psoriasis, but they may be exacerbating or triggering factors in some patients[6].

Despite these observations there is very little to suggest that bacterial infection is normally a cause of psoriasis. It just seems sometimes to be its trigger. Yeasts of the genus *Pityrosporum* have often been found in psoriatic skin lesions and skin scales. The organism is so often found in normal individuals that it is difficult to believe that it has a unique causal role; but since man and yeasts share many genes in common it remains possible that a yeast could yet be a trigger for psoriasis.

Clues from effective treatments

A large number of treatments for psoriasis have been tried and most are still in use. Tar preparations have been used for hundreds of years. Sunlight usually improves psoriasis, but is obviously of limited usefulness in most parts of the world. Its immunosuppressive and anti-proliferative effects can be greatly enhanced by psoralen drugs, but these drugs run the risk of causing skin cancer. Specific treatments of undoubted efficacy include glucocorticoid steroids and vitamin D analogues. Agents directly toxic to the proliferating skin cells include dithranol, methotrexate and retinoids, though all of these have potentially damaging side-effects. 'Keratinolytic' drugs (drugs that soften hard scale), such as salicylic acid, are useful. (They are the same drugs which are the main constituents of corn plasters.) Recently there has been interest in the use of peptides, chemicals built up from linked amino acids (see p. 85), but very much smaller than proteins. 'Peptide T' has been said to be effective in the treatment of psoriasis, possibly by stimulating release of another (larger) peptide hormone, somatostatin. These peptides act as chemical transmitters in nervous tissue – which perhaps suggests that stimulation of epidermal cells by such substances may underlie psoriasis.

Summary

Psoriasis is a common skin disease which in its mildest form produces scaly non-itchy patches on elbows and knees, but in its most violent form may involve large skin surfaces in raised and sometimes pustular lesions. It may also cause joint pains and deformities resembling those of rheumatoid arthritis.

Sufferers are not born with psoriasis, but are genetically predisposed to develop the condition when they encounter one of a number of possible environmental factors, especially infections. These act as triggers to set the disease off; but no consistently responsible trigger has yet been identified. Psychological factors may be important, but this is unproven. Many different genes seem able to confer susceptibility, but so far none has been recognised as invariably associated with psoriasis. Psoriasis is probably maintained by T-lymphocytes, which can by themselves carry or transmit the disease.

6

IRRITABLE BOWEL SYNDROME

Irritable bowel syndrome, often abbreviated to IBS, describes an extremely common intermittent disorder of bowel function. It is one of those medical mysteries like 'essential' hypertension (see Chapter 15) which is a diagnosis made by excluding other conditions. Unfortunately there is no test which proves the presence of IBS. Fortunately full investigation is neither necessary nor desirable in young people in whom the possibility of serious disease is remote.

Typically the disorder is episodic, with periods of remission to normal function. It may show itself in many different ways. Abdominal pain may occur at the time of passing a stool (defecation), or it may be associated with some change in bowel regularity. The pain may be severe, though it is more commonly mild. It may be felt anywhere in the abdomen, or even in the back. There is often increased slime (mucus) in the stool and sometimes gaseous abdominal distension. There may be a feeling after defecation that the bowel has not emptied properly, a situation given the neat description 'rectal dissatisfaction' (tenesmus). Some people have sub-classified IBS into abdominal pain + diarrhoea, abdominal pain + constipation, and abdominal pain with alternating diarrhoea and constipation. Chronic painless diarrhoea has been classified with IBS, but some people believe that it is an entirely separate condition.

IBS is nearly one and a half times commoner in women than in men. It has been reported from every part of the globe, more often in towns and cities than in the country. A recent survey suggested that 20% of the whole population of the UK will be affected by IBS at some stage in their lives, although only about half of them will consult a doctor. The incidence of new cases tends to decline with age. In the UK between 30% and 50% of all referrals by family doctors to hospital specialists are for patients suffering from the condition and 2½ million prescriptions are written each year for IBS.

IBS can be embarrassing and distressing. Its most disabling manifestation comprises frequent bowel emptying with occasional rectal incontinence. This can make patients frightened even to travel to work. Although most sufferers continue to work normally, IBS is almost the commonest reason for people taking time off work. Very frequent and urgent visits to the toilet are also socially disabling. Curiously, the urge to empty the bowel diminishes at night. Most sufferers from IBS enjoy undisturbed sleep. Diarrhoea interrupting sleep strongly suggests that something more serious is going on (e.g. inflammatory bowel disease – see Chapter 13).

Many IBS symptoms, especially pain, can occur in completely different conditions (e.g. endometriosis – see Chapter 11). Diverticular disease of the large bowel can be confused with IBS. This is perhaps not too surprising because it is even possible that abnormal gut movements in IBS may actually cause the out-pouchings in the large bowel (colon) which characterise diverticulosis. These can become inflamed, the condition known as diverticulitis. The early symptoms of cancer of the colon, before bleeding has been noted in the stool, are often the same as those of IBS. Thus middle-aged patients are commonly at some stage investigated by someone looking up the anus through a hollow tube with a light at the end, or with an instrument in which the image at the end is transmitted through closely-packed tiny glass rods (a flexible colonoscope). In older patients, in whom cancer is a greater risk, an X-ray of the lower bowel is usually also taken after flushing in a 'barium enema' which contains barium sulphate. This insoluble material is opaque to X-rays.

Cause

There is no general agreement about the cause of IBS, though most evidence suggests that the symptoms are due to defective or incoordinated movements of the gut. No structural abnormalities can be discovered by investigation during life, or even at post-mortem examination. So the mystery remains. What causes the abnormal gut movements?

Control of gut motility

The gullet, stomach, and small and large intestines (Fig. 10) are not passive tubes. Rings of coordinated contraction in all these organs slowly propel gut contents from the mouth towards the anus. Fig. 11 is a record of pressure changes in a section of human small intestine. Contraction waves come along every minute or so and get alternately weaker and stronger over a 90-minute cycle. Since the gut is some 30 feet long when stretched out and since the waves of contraction come along quite slowly it may take a day or more for the residues of

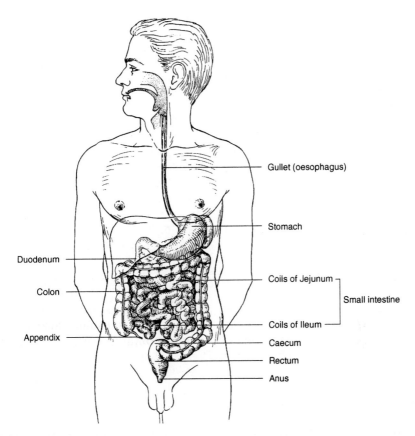

Gullet (oesophagus)

Stomach

Duodenum

Coils of Jejunum ⎤
⎥ Small intestine
Colon

Coils of Ileum ⎦

Appendix

Caecum

Rectum

Anus

Figure 10 Diagram of the main structures of the gut. The stomach leads into the duodenum, which itself leads into coils of jejunum and ileum – all comprising the 'small intestine'. The ileum leads into the 'large intestine' which comprises the colon, the appendix, the caecum and the rectum, before terminating at the anus.

ingested food to be excreted. Contraction waves are generated by a network of nerves running in the gut wall. These are 'hard-wired' into the gut itself. The network, described as a nerve 'plexus' (Latin: braid/plait) can almost be regarded as an independent brain which sends nerve messages up to the head and receives nerve messages in return to control gut movements. Slow moving contraction waves called 'migrating motor complexes' moving in the appropriate normal direction can be seen in lengths of animal colon isolated outside the body[1].

Although such coordinated movements can take place in isolated gut, overriding control is exerted by the nervous system and by local

51

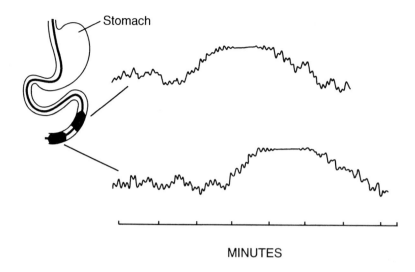

Stomach

MINUTES

Figure 11 Waves of contraction moving slowly along the upper human small intestine, recorded as pressure changes in two fluid-filled balloons in the jejunum. The upper trace shows pressure changes in the upper balloon (the one nearest the stomach). The lower trace is from a second balloon a few inches lower down the gut. Pressure increase is shown by upward deflection of the trace. The maximum pressure comes about a minute later in the lower trace. (From an original record obtained by Michael Atkinson).

or circulating chemical factors. Nervous control is exerted through the so-called autonomic nervous system (see p. 32), which is mostly outside conscious control. The two main divisions of the autonomic nervous system have opposite effects on the gut. Excessive activity of sympathetic nerves slows gut movements down and causes constipation, while excessive activity of parasympathetic nerves causes colicky pain and diarrhoea. It also increases gut secretions. Many circulating or locally-secreted chemicals (hormones) mimic some actions of the central nervous system. The multiplicity of factors influencing gut motility makes systematic study of IBS very difficult.

Possible role of infection

IBS often begins as persistent diarrhoea months after an attack of infective gastroenteritis. All of us have experienced attacks of infective diarrhoea, just lasting a few days. Such symptoms are usually attributed, correctly, to 'food poisoning'. Most such attacks clear up on their own, so doctors seldom investigate them by sending a stool specimen to the lab. A low-grade gut infection with some as yet

52

unidentified disease-producing organism (a 'pathogen') might be the trigger which starts off IBS. Such an infection might involve a virus, bacterium or protozoon.

Viruses are minute complex chemical structures which can only survive and replicate inside the cells of the body. They are usually parasites: that is, their replication and activity is damaging to the infected cell. Several common viruses disturb bowel function, especially in their early invasive stage (e.g. rotavirus, astrovirus and Norwalk virus). Bacteria are larger but still microscopic single-cell organisms which in most cases have some ability to survive and multiply outside body cells. Many different bacteria can infect the bowel (e.g. salmonella species are common causes of so-called 'food poisoning' as well as of typhoid fever; *Vibrio cholerae* causes the serious tropical disease cholera). Protozooa are single-cell organisms, larger than bacteria, with a definite nucleus. *Giardia lamblia* is a protozoon which is a common cause of mild but tiresome diarrhoea. It is usually acquired by drinking infected water. *Entamoeba histolytica* is another example of a protozoon which causes diarrhoea and much more severe inflammation of the bowel. Infection of the bowel by fungi has been looked for in IBS but not found. When 'thrush' (the fungal infection candidiasis) involves the anus there has usually been some loss of normal immunological function (e.g. because of AIDS – see p. 26). However, unless one of these infections persists in the bowel wall, for which there is no evidence in IBS, it is not clear why the symptoms should continue.

One suggestion has been that there might be a disturbed balance between different bacteria within the colon itself. There have been reports that antibiotics given to women before gynaecological operations such as hysterectomy may trigger IBS. Many different bacteria can be found in the colon, including harmless and protective bacteria (e.g. some of the lactobacilli) and harmful ones such as certain 'entero-pathogenic' (gut harming) strains of *Escherichia coli (E. coli)*. Current estimates are that there are 300 different species of bacteria living together in the large bowel and that there are some 500 million living bacteria present in each ounce of intestinal contents. Some physicians get IBS patients to swallow cultures of certain specific bacteria (e.g. *Lactobacillus plantarum*) in the hope that 'good' bacteria will drive out harmful ones. Eating live yoghurt is often recommended. But in view of the enormous variety of different bacteria present, such an approach seems a bit naive. The large bowel has the property of 'colonisation resistance', largely the result of immunological defence mechanisms. These protect against damaging bacteria taking hold, but make it more difficult to change the microbial environment or indeed to restore it after the inappropriate use of antibiotics.

Possible role of malabsorption

Another possibility is that sufferers don't absorb certain sugars properly (e.g. fructose, lactose and sorbitol). In some cases this could be due to relative lack of a digestive enzyme (e.g. of lactase, which is necessary to split lactose before it can be absorbed). Accumulation of undigested sugars might perhaps lead to undue fermentation in the colon and local irritability of the bowel wall. But careful comparisons of IBS patients with normal people have not revealed any failure of absorptive function in IBS. None the less, patients sometimes report that eating sugary things produces symptoms or makes existing symptoms worse.

Food allergy or intolerance

IBS may overlap in its symptoms with the syndrome of intolerance to gluten, a protein found in wheat. Gluten intolerance of severe degree causes 'coeliac disease' which is often associated with diarrhoea. Some patients who don't have the gut changes which characterise coeliac disease have reported improvement in their IBS symptoms by avoiding wheat gluten.

Diarrhoea in children is well-known to be sometimes associated with intolerance to cows' milk. It is less well known that chronic constipation can also be due to cows' milk. It is not known whether in adults cows' milk plays a part in producing the symptoms of IBS in some people, but the possibility might repay further investigation.

Nervous and psychological factors

Many investigators (perhaps most) believe that psychological factors are important[2]. Sufferers from IBS have more often experienced severe anxiety or depression in the past than people without IBS. Hypnosis or self-hypnosis has benefited some patients. Sufferers often complain of undue fatigue. Symptoms sometimes overlap with those of chronic fatigue syndrome (see Chapter 12). Patients with IBS seem to have a reduced pain threshold to distension of their gut by balloons[3]. An interesting recent report[4] is that IBS sufferers spend more time in the phase of sleep associated with dreaming and rapid eye movements (REM) than comparable people without IBS. This would fit in with the idea that sufferers have a built-in (intrinsic) alteration in central nervous system function.

Emotions can have profound effects on gut function because the nerve networks in the walls of the gut are connected to the brain. When we experience an attack of diarrhoea in a frightening situation the brain has sent messages to the large bowel via the autonomic nervous system. Isolated rear gunners in bombers during the 1939–45 war were well-known to be troubled by rectal incontinence. Certain local chemicals which are 'neurotransmitters'[*] can modify and sensitise the connections between brain and bowel. Serotonin is one such substance, antagonists of which are being actively investigated for treatment of IBS[5]. The trouble is that such treatment reduces bowel motility. It risks converting uncomfortable diarrhoea into equally troublesome constipation.

Many investigations have been made of gut movements in IBS. They have been notably inconsistent, though the rate of transit of food through the gut has usually been found to be increased.

If sufferers from undue anxiety or stress are more likely than normal people to complain of IBS symptoms, does this mean that the cause lies in the brain? Not necessarily. Maybe a primary disorder in the gut itself is sending nerve messages to the brain which result in feelings of anxiety. Furthermore lots of people have IBS without any evidence of psychological disorder. Many investigators are not convinced that IBS is a manifestation of an inner psychological disturbance, even though IBS is one of those conditions in which there may be a good response to so-called 'placebos' – treatments masquerading as active drugs when they are not. Perhaps the cause should not be regarded as psychological, but rather as representing some defect in the way the brain processes information coming from sensory nerves running from the bowel to the brain, somehow leading to uncoordinated muscle movements of the gut wall.

Apart from serotonin, many other chemicals influence gut movements and might be released from nerve endings in the gut walls (e.g. acetylcholine and vaso-active intestinal peptide). Undoubtedly IBS symptoms are made worse by the so-called 'affective' psychological disorders (those involving emotional disturbance). But they are probably not *caused* by them because IBS symptoms usually appear before the psychiatric ones. Severe IBS symptoms might, obviously, so disturb someone's life that the symptoms themselves might initiate an affective disorder. (This is one of the many situations in medicine and psychiatry where a 'chicken or egg' problem arises). So far there is no universal agreement about either the cause or the best treatment of

---

[*] A neurotransmitter is a chemical released locally from a nerve ending which modifies the receptive state of another adjacent excitable nerve cell. More than 40 different neurotransmitters have been recognised.

IBS, though drugs which relax the specialised muscle tissue in the bowel wall can help a bit (e.g. peppermint oil, mebeverine or alverine). Diarrhoea can be treated by various drugs which reduce gut movements (e.g. loperamide or codeine). Constipation may be improved by a high fibre diet, though this is disputed. If certain foods seem to be triggers, they should obviously be avoided.

I am very suspicious of psychological explanations for bodily symptoms. As a general physician ('internist') I have seen many people complaining of apparently inexplicable symptoms such as abdominal pain, indigestion, bowel disturbance, loss of appetite, loss of weight, low-grade fever, chronic fatigue and dizzy attacks, in whom a physical cause eventually became apparent. My best guess is that in the case of most otherwise normal people with IBS the cause lies in what they have been eating. Food may be contaminated with infectious material. One thinks of the frequent salmonella scares. I think that it is quite likely that an infecting bowel bacterium, one of the *E. coli* variants, for example, might achieve an uneasy half-symbiotic/half-parasitic relationship with its host, causing IBS symptoms whenever it gained the upper hand. I am also intrigued by the potential rivalry between 'good' and 'bad' bacteria in the gut. There is, of course, every reason to expect that someone's emotional state can aggravate, modify or suppress IBS caused in the first instance by food intolerance or allergy. Man shares many genes in common with lower animals and plants. Each gene from, say, yeast codes for a different protein. Foreign proteins are often the triggers for allergic reactions. So there are good theoretical reasons for supposing that vegetable products could well act as low-grade 'allergens' (substances able to provoke an allergic reaction). People in developed countries eat such an enormous variety of different foods that it may be very difficult for an affected individual to identify one specific dietary item as a precipitant of IBS symptoms. Tinned foods in particular contain many different chemicals as preservatives, artificial flavouring or colouring. True food allergy is rare. Careful studies suggest that it may affect 1.4% of the adult population and between 5% and 7% of children[6]. But IBS might yet be brought about by a low-grade allergic reaction only affecting gut movements, without causing gut inflammation.

The symptoms of IBS can be so severe that some victims have been prepared to have an abdominal operation to allow a full-thickness specimen of their bowel wall to be examined. Preliminary results have been fascinating[7]. They suggest that although the superficial layers of the gut (the epithelium) always look normal under the microscope, the deeper layers may contain infiltrating lymphocytes, suggesting that chronic inflammation of the bowel wall might underlie IBS. If these results are confirmed they could provide a focus for further research.

Whatever the main cause of IBS eventually proves to be, its discoverer will earn a great debt of gratitude from the many sufferers from this very common condition.

Summary

Irritable bowel syndrome is a common condition of unknown cause which can cause abdominal pain and bowel disturbance. There is often increased slime in the stool and sometimes gaseous abdominal distension. There may be a feeling after defecation that the bowel has not emptied properly. IBS has been sub-classified into abdominal pain + diarrhoea, pain + constipation, and pain with alternating diarrhoea and constipation. Although there seems to be evidence of a disturbance of normal gut motility, numerous investigations have been notably inconsistent, though there is some new evidence for an underlying inflammatory process. Perhaps something in ingested food, possibly a low-grade bacterial infection, might be its cause.

The symptoms may be augmented by psychological disturbance; but psychological disturbance may also arise from the bowel symptoms themselves. It is often difficult for the physician, let alone the patient, to sort the problem out.

7

CLUBBING OF THE FINGERS

Doctors describe 'clubbing' of the fingers as a 'physical sign'. Clubbing is not a disease, but it is a marker for a lot of different diseases. It was first observed by Hippocrates in the 5th century BC. He noted that in severe lung infections with pus collecting in the chest the fingernails became curved and warm, especially at their tips. We now recognise the earliest manifestation of clubbing as increased thickness of the nail bed and of the soft tissues below it. The most objective criterion is that clubbing is present when the depth (i.e. top to bottom thickness) of the last segment of the index finger (measurement A in Fig. 12) is the same or greater than the depth of the terminal finger joint (measurement B). The finger pulp is swollen and infiltrated with white blood cells. When clubbing is severe the fingers really look like small clubs. The finger-tip

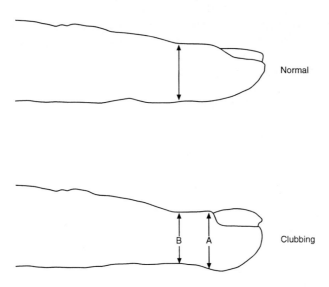

Diagram of measurements to define clubbing of the index finger

Figure 12   A normal and a typical 'clubbed' index finger, viewed from the side. Clubbing is present when measurement A is the same or greater than measurement B.

blood capillaries are dilated and the number of blood vessels is increased. Most authors have reported that blood flow through the fingers is also increased.

When clubbing is severe it may be associated with changes in the small bones of the limbs, especially wrist bones. These may become painful and swollen: a condition known as 'hypertrophic osteoarthropathy' (Greek: 'hyper' = excessive; 'troph-' = growth; 'osteo-' = bone; 'arthro-' = joint; 'path-' = suffering). There is new bone formation at the distal ends of long bones, especially the lower arm bones at the wrists, which may be hot and painful, with increased blood flow through new blood vessels.

Association of clubbing with disease

1 Clubbing can (rarely) occur in families as a 'dominant' characteristic[*] and even sporadically without evidence of any gross underlying disease or anatomical abnormality. However, in most cases it is pathological. In many situations it is a sinister physical sign.
2 It is always present in 'blue babies' and also in blue adults. (The description 'cyanotic' simply comes from Greek: 'kyan-' = blue.) Such people are born with some abnormality of the heart causing unoxygenated blue blood coming from the veins in the body to be pumped straight into the systemic arteries, without passing through the lungs. The shunt is definitely the cause of clubbing in these circumstances because clubbing disappears if the shunt is surgically closed.
3 Clubbing also occurs in some diffuse lung diseases associated with poor oxygenation of the blood, in which there is a right to left shunt of blood through underventilated parts of the lungs.
4 Generalised clubbing, of fingers and often toes as well, is recognised as characteristic of long-standing subacute bacterial endocarditis (a blood-borne infection of the heart valves). It disappears after successful treatment of the infection.
5 Localised clubbing, affecting only one upper or lower limb has been observed when there has been severe infection in an arterial graft in a large artery supplying that limb. In such cases the localised arterial infection has clearly caused the clubbing. It disappears in those cases in which the infection can be eradicated or the graft replaced.
6 Some long-standing infections of the lungs and chest cavity can

[*] 'Dominant' means that a child can inherit the condition even if only one parent has it.

cause clubbing without necessarily being associated with low arterial oxygen content and blue blood. Examples are lung abscess, empyema (pus in the chest), cystic fibrosis and bronchiectasis. The causal relationship here also seems clear, because clubbing has often been noted to disappear after successful treatment of the underlying condition (e.g. draining pus from an empyema).

7 Clubbing has been noted to accompany chronic liver disease and to disappear when cirrhosis has been treated by liver transplantation[1]. The liver disease must therefore have been the immediate underlying cause.

8 Tumours of the lungs and lung linings are also often associated with clubbing. This can occur even if the blood is well oxygenated. Clubbing may disappear if a cancer is successfully removed.

9 Clubbing is well-known to occur sometimes in chronic inflammatory diseases of the gut (especially Crohn's disease: see Chapter 13).

Previous theories to explain clubbing

The number and apparent diversity of recognised causes or associations of clubbing at first sight make any single hypothesis of pathogenesis untenable. Let me begin by concentrating on the most consistent occurrence of clubbing: in cyanotic congenital heart disease. In this situation large amounts of blue (deoxygenated) venous blood coming to the heart pass directly into the systemic arterial circulation without going through the lungs. This suggests that as blood passes through the lungs of normal people, either a clubbing-producing factor is removed from the blood, or a clubbing-preventing factor is added to the blood. The second possibility seems unlikely since there are no obvious pulmonary secretory glands or tissues. Most authors have therefore speculated on the possible nature of a clubbing-producing factor which normal lungs remove. But none is yet generally accepted as a plausible candidate.

A large number of circulating substances have been studied. I have summarised all these in a recent review[2]. In each case there has been considerable overlap of blood concentration of the suspect material between clubbed and unclubbed patients. None of the previous theories explain why clubbing should occur beyond infected large arteries or arterial grafts, nor its common occurrence in sub-acute bacterial endocarditis. Venous blood, low in oxygen and high in carbon dioxide (the waste gas), will obviously lower the blood oxygen and raise blood carbon dioxide concentrations if it gets into the arteries unchanged. But these gas changes in the blood definitely do not cause clubbing. People can be almost at death's door with long-standing airways obstruction causing gross cyanosis without becoming clubbed. Indeed, when clubbing is seen in chronic lung disease and respiratory failure, an associated cancer of the lung is often found.

For at least 50 years reviewers have speculated that a potent active substance produced by tissue metabolism, but normally destroyed during the passage of blood through the pulmonary capillaries, might be the cause of clubbing. All such theories failed because no appropriate or plausible factor could be identified. A new approach was needed.

The megakaryocyte/platelet clump hypothesis

John Martin and I proposed, in 1987, an entirely new theory: that particulate matter rather than a soluble factor was the cause of clubbing[3]. This idea was stimulated by recent work on megakaryocyte and platelet physiology. Megakaryocytes (Greek: 'mega' = large; 'kary-' = nut; 'cyt-' = hollow/cell) are large cells produced in the bone marrow. Each megakaryocyte breaks up into many hundreds of platelets. Platelets are tiny cells with a vital role in blood clotting. (Aspirin protects against coronary thrombosis mainly by reducing the stickiness of platelets.) Megakaryocytes are relatively abundant in mixed venous blood but scarce in arterial blood, whereas platelets are more abundant in arterial than in venous blood. Calculations about the sizes of platelets and megakaryocytes and the relative numbers of each led to the proposition that most platelets are produced in the lungs, in lung capillaries, by physical fragmentation of megarkaryocytes*.

Normal lung capillaries are narrow. Suspended particulate matter of average diameter greater than 20–50 microns (three to seven times the diameter of a red blood cell) are too big to pass through normal lung capillaries. Consequently only the denuded nuclei of megakaryocytes are seen in arterial blood, together with clumps of platelets. Megakaryocytes can often be observed apparently stuck in lung capillaries when lungs are examined after death.

---

* I chanced upon John Martin's fascinating work and calculations when I was browsing around posters at a meeting of the British Medical Research Society several years ago. Posters are a popular way of communicating new scientific information at meetings. The poster I saw was headed provocatively 'Platelets are made in the lungs'. I had always believed that platelets were made in the bone marrow. It took me ten minutes' careful study to realise what John and his colleagues were getting at. The meeting led directly to our original publication. It's always worth looking at posters at scientific meetings!

A large right to left shunt of blood such as blue babies have will necessarily let megakaryocytes themselves, large fragments of megakar- yocytes, and large platelet clumps straight through into the systemic arterial circulation. This is confirmed by observations that the size distribution of platelets and platelet aggregates in congenital heart disease with a right to left shunt of blood is exactly what would be expected of the passage of abnormally large particles into the arterial blood. Large particles in flowing blood tend to travel in a central (axial) stream. They will therefore preferentially tend to land up in the tips of the fingers and toes, which is where clubbing occurs.

Platelet-derived growth factor: a potential clubbing-producing factor

Platelets and megakaryocytes contain growth-stimulating chemicals, one of which is 'platelet-derived growth factor' (PDGF). Although the three forms of this small polypeptide were first recognised in platelets, they have since been found in many other cells and tissues. PDGF is a general growth promoter of connective tissues. It increases blood vessel permeability.

Especially in one of its forms (known as '-BB') it stimulates the growth of new blood vessels and attracts white cells out of the blood- stream. It plays a part in the inflammatory response. Thus the impac- tion of a megakaryocyte or a large clump of platelets in a fingertip could locally release high concentrations of PDGF. This material has effects which could account for all the pathological changes of clubbing (e.g. increased thickness of the nail bed and pulp, accumula- tion of excess tissue fluid and increased blood vessel growth). I shall discuss arterial growth factors further in Chapter 21.

Another potential similar factor present in platelets is 'transforming growth factor beta-1'(TGFβ1). This material can be detected in higher concentrations in the blood of patients with clubbing than in those without. We do not at present know the relative importance of PDGF and TGFβ1. They might both be involved in producing the pathological changes of clubbing.

Conditions explicable by the megakaryocyte/platelet clump hypothesis

The hypothesis obviously accounts for the occurrence of clubbing in the presence of gross right to left shunts (Category 2, above); but it also accounts well for clubbing in Category 3, in which blood travels through distended pulmonary blood vessels. When people with pre-existent clubbing move to live at high altitudes, clubbing has been seen to increase. This can be logically explained because the increased flow of blood through the lungs must involve dilation of the blood vessels of the lungs. This would make it more likely that megakaryocytes and platelet clumps would pass through unchanged. In addition, megakaryocytes exposed to low oxygen concentrations may increase their production of PDGF. In respect of Category 4 above, loose platelet clumps form on heart valves in sub-acute bacterial endocarditis. Platelets are known to clump in a similar way in damaged and ballooned-out arterial walls ('aneurysms') and in infected arterial grafts (Category 5, above).

Chronic inflammatory conditions of the lungs and pleura

Although clubbing is rare in chronic lung infections which do not produce pus (such as tuberculosis), it is common in lung abscess, empyema, bronchiectasis and cystic fibrosis (Category 6, above). In these conditions it is reasonable to assume that in the neighbourhood of the infection there will be dilated blood vessels. In addition, inflammatory conditions of this sort may predispose to platelet aggregates and clots in veins draining the inflamed areas. Such infections might be relevant both to Categories 3 and 4, above.

Clubbing in liver disease

At first sight, clubbing in liver disease (Category 7, above) is not explained by the megakaryocyte hypothesis. The diseased liver must be at fault, because clubbing has been observed to improve or disappear after successful liver transplantation, and to reappear if a liver transplant is rejected. However, the lung circulation is abnormal in severe liver disease. Patients are sometimes blue and have even been wrongly diagnosed as having congenital heart disease with a right to left shunt. In some cases of chronic liver disease (cirrhosis) many small abnormal connections between arteries and veins in the lungs have been shown on X-ray or by other means.

Tests of the lung circulation have been made in man by injecting into an arm vein radioactive particles of different sizes (usually technetium-labelled macroaggregates of albumin). Because of their radioactivity these labelled particles can be followed to the lungs to find whether the particles get through or stick there. In severe liver disease there are abnormally large lung blood vessels which allow particles of 20–50 microns diameter to pass through. Even more convincing is a report of the effects of liver transplantation carried out to treat a patient whose liver was damaged by 'biliary cirrhosis', a rare but very serious disease. The clubbing previously present disappeared at the same time that the abnormal shunts closed. Particles larger than 20 microns diameter could no longer pass through the lung circulation[1].

Lung tumours associated with clubbing

Lung cancers are often associated with clubbing (Category 8, above). Clubbing has also been observed in tumours of the pleura (the lining membrane of the lungs). It has been observed to disappear after successful treatment (e.g. with radiotherapy or chemotherapy). In these situations, the tumour itself may supply a vascular shunt conveying blood from right to left heart without being filtered through pulmonary capillaries (Category 3, above). This could therefore provide at least part of the explanation for clubbing in Category 8. In addition, lung tumours may themselves produce growth factors. They may also be associated with larger than normal megakaryocytes and an increased platelet count. The relatively frequent association of hypertrophic osteoarthropathy with lung tumours suggests that factors additional to a local right to left shunt may be involved.

Clubbing in other conditions

There is not much information about the lung circulation in other conditions (e.g. Category 9, above). The platelet excess often observed in such conditions might have something to do with the clubbing sometimes seen in Crohn's disease (see Chapter 13). I shall discuss later (in Chapter 18) the possible relevance of gut factors to the lung circulation.

To summarise, although the reason for some of the associations remains uncertain, the megakaryocyte/platelet clump hypothesis provides an explanation for most causes of clubbing. It is not disproved by any currently available evidence.

Pathological support for the megakaryocyte/platelet hypothesis

A preliminary report by Stephen Fox and his colleagues[4] gave strong support to the hypothesis. At the time of post-mortem examination they looked through the microscope at the nail beds of 24 unclubbed patients and 7 patients who had died with clubbing present. The latter included four cases of lung cancer and one of fibrosing alveolitis, all with unequivocal clubbing, and two cases with mild or early clubbing.

Two specimens were taken from each cadaver and stained with specific dyes to show platelet aggregates in nail-bed capillaries. All five patients with notable clubbing had numerous tiny aggregated platelet clots (microthrombi) in their nail-bed capillaries; the two with mild or early clubbing had fewer platelet microthrombi. By contrast, in only 4 out of 25 controls were 'very occasional platelet and whole blood microthrombi identified'. Dr Fox has kindly allowed me to mention two of his further (unpublished) observations on nail-bed punch specimens taken during life from two patients with clubbing of unknown cause. In both of these numerous platelet microthrombi were identified in nail-bed capillaries.

I found these observations, independently confirming exactly what the hypothesis had predicted, immensely exciting. In an ideal world a scientist first identifies a problem, thinks how it might be explained and finally carries out the appropriate observation or experiment him- or herself. Some people deride those who just propose hypotheses and go no further. This is unfair. The failure to pursue a particular line of investigation may certainly be due to laziness, but maybe the necessary techniques or facilities were not available at the time. There have been many successful theoretical predictions in physics which were not immediately testable but which would not have been later examined if the hypothesis or prediction had not been made in the first place.

Objections to the megakaryocyte/platelet clump hypothesis

The strongest potential criticism is that the large right to left shunt present before birth in the 'fetus' (the technical term for a baby as yet unborn) is not accompanied by clubbing. (This objection, of course, applies with equal force to all current theories which ascribe clubbing to something carried in the blood and normally inactivated during passage through the lungs.) Megakaryocytes are present in near normal numbers in fetal bone-marrow in the last months of pregnancy. There are about the same numbers of platelets in the blood of the newborn baby as in the adult, but more megakaryocytes in fetal arterial than in venous umbilical cord blood. Megakaryocytes undoubtedly populate the systemic arterial blood of the fetus. Many must inevitably arrive at the fingertips. Since newborn babies are not normally clubbed, is the hypothesis wrong?

Fetal platelet function

Although they work well as far as blood clotting is concerned, platelets of the fetus and the newborn are far less reactive than platelets of the adult. Platelets in fetal or newborn blood do not clump together normally. There is an 'intrinsically defective release reaction which may reflect immaturity of membrane structure'. They have a 'defect in the release of their dense-body contents, most marked in response to adrenaline'[5]. All these markers of platelet immaturity disappear within a few days of birth. I cannot find any information about the content or release of PDGF by fetal or newborn platelets. But in view of the many measures of immaturity already identified, especially the inability of fetal platelets to release a number of substances when activated, it would be most surprising if PDGF function was not also reduced. In evolutionary development this would obviously be desirable, otherwise there could be unrestrained and random growth stimulation at many sites of impaction of fetal megakaryocytes, which are in high concentration in fetal arterial blood.

Hypertrophic osteoarthropathy

People with HOA have almost invariably severe clubbing, but we do not know if it has a different cause. HOA is relatively common in cancer of the lung, being found in about 10% of cases, though it is less common and much less florid in people with cyanotic congenital heart disease. One difference could be in megakaryocyte function. I have reviewed elsewhere reasons for the slightly different predisposition of various diseases to clubbing and HOA[2].

Unsolved problems

A good hypothesis should not only be testable and falsifiable: it should spawn further work. One obvious subject needing study is the occurrence of congenital and familial clubbing, in the absence of discoverable pathology. Do such patients have distended pulmonary vessels or multiple small connections between pulmonary arteries and veins, as in liver disease? Is megakaryocyte and platelet physiology normal, especially in respect of PDGF production and release? In inflammatory bowel disease with clubbing are similar changes found in the lung blood vessels as have already been shown in severe liver disease accompanied by clubbing? Are platelet PDGF production and release affected?

Clubbing is unusual in long-standing airways obstruction, such as occurs in severe chronic bronchitis. The hypothesis would therefore predict that despite the low oxygen in the blood there would not be significantly enlarged shunt channels. This prediction has not so far been specially looked for. As I have already mentioned, the hypothesis also predicts, in comparison with the situation in adults, that fetal platelets should have reduced PDGF content or impaired PDGF release, or that fetal tissue PDGF receptor function should be impaired. Nothing appears to be known as yet about any of these possibilities. None the less, on a personal note, I have been delighted by the striking success of the original hypothesis. It has not so far been disproved and has provided a plausible explanation for clubbing in the great majority of situations.

Summary

'Clubbing' of the fingers (and toes) is the name given to swelling of the tips of the digits and curvature of the nails. It has been recognised for more than 2000 years as a physical sign which can occur in many different diseases, including pus in the chest and blue (cyanotic) congenital heart disease. Many different explanations have been put forward over the years.

According to the most recent and so far cautiously accepted explanation, clubbing may be due to the impaction of megakaryocytes and platelet clumps in the fingers and toes, to which these particles have passed in an axial stream of blood travelling from the heart to the tissues. A pilot post-mortem study has confirmed the expected findings in nail beds of people with finger clubbing. It seems likely that at the site of impaction platelet-derived growth factor is released. This material is a general growth promoter. It is known to have effects which include all the pathological changes recognised to occur in clubbed digits. Other platelet-derived factors may also play a part.

In congenital heart disease with a right to left shunt of blood large particles can pass directly from bone-marrow to the main arterial circulation without getting broken up in the lungs, as they normally are. In sub-acute bacterial endocarditis and in arterial aneurysms or infected arterial grafts, platelet clumps form locally on heart valves or on the damaged arterial wall. Then they become detached and pass peripherally. This mechanism accounts well for localised clubbing. In those lung diseases in which clubbing is common there may be not only local shunting of blood through abnormal right to left connections, but also local aggregation of platelets. In some cases there is also altered platelet function. In severe liver disease, clubbing can be accounted for by multiple small artery-to-vein shunts in the lungs.

Clubbing might be expected in the newborn (because blood largely bypasses the lungs during fetal life) but is not found. The likeliest explanation is that fetal platelet PDGF release is undeveloped or inhibited, as are many other fetal platelet release functions: but this matter has not so far been investigated.

'Hypertrophic osteoarthropathy' is a painful disease of the ends of long bones. It is usually associated with severe clubbing. A mild degree of this condition can be found in congenital heart disease with right to left shunts, but its special occurrence and severity in certain diseases suggests that some factor additional to a right to left shunt of blood may be operating.

8

RHEUMATOID ARTHRITIS

Rheumatoid arthritis (RA) is one of the commonest disabling diseases. A strict definition is impossible because its symptoms, signs and findings on investigation overlap with many other conditions. Because of this, the incidence of the disease (the number of new cases per year) has to be inferred by comparisons of prevalence estimates (the numbers of the population affected by the disease) made at different points in time. Such comparisons suggest that at least 2 in every 10,000 people will develop definite rheumatoid arthritis each year. At any time at least 1 in every 100 of the population will be suffering from the condition. This estimate of prevalence has been made using strict criteria for diagnosis. Everyday observation suggests that the real prevalence is much higher than this. Many mild cases are undoubtedly overlooked or not recorded. Although RA is not thought of as a fatal disease, about 1000 deaths per year in the UK are attributed to it, though many of these are misadventures with anti-rheumatoid therapy. Smoking is associated with RA in men and may make the symptoms worse, but it seems to have no effect on RA in women. Schizophrenia is negatively associated with RA: i.e. if someone has schizophrenia he or she is considerably less likely than the average person to develop RA. The reasons for both these strange observations are unknown.

Bone is hard; but bone surfaces in joints are covered with cartilage, which is smooth and relatively soft. Lubrication is supplied by 'hyaluronan', a matrix material which enables joint surfaces to slide over one another without causing damage. Hyaluronan is produced by the 'synovium', which is a thin layer of cells (a membrane) lining the joints. There are several features common to most cases of RA. One is that the synovium is mainly involved. In RA there is widespread inflammation of many synovial membranes, especially in the hands. The knuckles of the fingers (the metacarpo-phalangeal (MCP) joints) and the first finger joints (the proximal inter-phalangeal (PIP) joints) are particularly affected and swell up (Fig. 13). The wrists, the knees and sometimes other joints may also be involved. The disease is roughly symmetrical in its manifestations: i.e. if a particular joint on

71

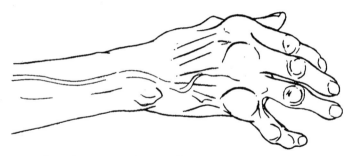

Figure 13 Drawing of a hand seriously affected by rheumatoid arthritis. Note that the knuckles (the metacarpo-phalangeal joints) are severely swollen and the fingers are deviated in the opposite direction to the thumb (so-called 'ulnar deviation'). There is also considerable wasting of the small (intrinsic) hand and finger muscles.

one side is affected, the same joint on the other side is almost always involved, to a similar extent. There is also the formation of 'pannus' (Latin: cloth), a destructive tumour-like growth within joints caused by synovium invading cartilage and acquiring a blood supply of its own. This restricts joint movement and further damages joint surfaces. Another rather constant feature is the appearance of hard, usually painless, nodules under the skin of the elbows and forearms.

The bone around affected joints is often weakened or destroyed. One possible reason for this is the behaviour of certain white blood cells which accumulate in the synovial cavities of affected joints. When they are cultured outside the body they can aggregate and turn into single large cells with several nuclei. These have all the characteristics of 'osteoclasts', which are specialised cells able to remove bone. The same thing happening in RA probably explains the bone destruction which is always found around severely affected joints.

Rheumatoid factors and complement

'Rheumatoid factors' are specialised antibodies known as autoantibodies[*1]. These chemicals react with some of the body's own normal constituents – hence the term 'auto' (self). Rheumatoid factors are usually present in the blood in RA, though RA can occur without rheumatoid factors being present and rheumatoid factors can be found without RA. In general, rheumatoid factors are associated with severe rather than mild disease. These circulating antibodies are produced by specialised cells in lymph glands and tissues, the so-called 'B-lympho-

---

[*] Technically, these react with the 'fragment crystallisable' (Fc) part of immunoglobulin G.

cytes'. These comprise some of the non-pigmented white cells of the blood and seem to be particularly involved in RA. B-lymphocytes produce specialised Y-shaped protein molecules. The variable parts of these molecules can take on many shapes, allowing them to combine with, and in effect wrap up, many different foreign chemical molecules, making them harmless. In RA, unfortunately, there seems to be an abnormal survival and excess of B-lymphocytes, which attack synovial membranes and seem to treat them as foreign material.

An antigen-antibody complex or an antibody can set in motion (activate) a complicated sequence of linked chemical changes in certain constituents of the blood plasma (the fluid part not containing any cells). The chemicals concerned are all proteins or large polypeptides, predominantly made in the liver and present in the form of inactive enzyme precursors. Collectively they are referred to as 'complement'. More than 25 separate complement proteins have been identified. These can make an amplifying cascade of enzyme reactions reminiscent of the amplifying cascade of reactions involved in blood clotting. The so-called 'classical' complement pathway is activated by antigen-antibody complexes. A slower 'alternative' pathway can be activated by antibody alone or directly by invading microbes. Recently a third activation pathway has been discovered to be associated with 'mannose-binding protein'.

Complement damages the membranes of cells perceived as foreign or coats the cells with a combination of complement proteins, forming the so-called 'membrane attack complex' (MAC). The body's defensive white blood cells then swallow up the coated cells. At different stages of the cascade of chemical reactions cytokines are released. Complement activation and cytokine release play an important part in causing tissue damage in conditions such as RA. The complement system is also involved in hypersensitivity and most immune reactions[2]. It makes potential targets for the suppression of damaging reactions. Despite this, complement effects are overall beneficial. Deficiencies of complement factors can have serious consequences. For example, a genetic defect in mannose-binding protein predisposes to particularly severe bacterial infections (e.g. those causing meningitis).

T-lymphocytes and cytokines

There is involvement of so-called 'T-lymphocytes' in RA[3]. These cells are directly concerned with immune defences against direct attacks on body cells rather than (indirectly) with the circulating defensive antibodies produced by the B-lymphocytes. T-lymphocytes have been identified in rheumatoid-affected joint tissues. Arthritis can readily be induced in rats which have been first primed to respond to a foreign chemical antigen and then given injections of the same material into a joint. Although this sounds unlikely to occur naturally, defensive macrophage cells can carry foreign antigens into joint cavities.

At present the precise role of T-lymphocytes in RA is uncertain, though they are probably involved in the release of damaging cytokines. Treatment of patients with an antibody to the cytokine called 'tumour necrosis factor alpha' (TNFα) has been spectacularly successful in relieving RA patients of pain and disability. Unfortunately the improvement does not last long because the anti-TNFα antibodies are soon recognised by the body as foreign chemicals. The body then produces antibodies which inactivate them. This is unfortunately the story in many of the treatments for RA which have been tried over the years. Some patients initially improve, but problems appear with longer-term therapy. However, newer synthetic and less immunogenic materials are coming along. In addition, prolonged relief of symptoms in rheumatoid arthritis is now being obtained by giving anti-TNFα antibodies combined with the anti-cell-dividing drug methotrexate, which decreases the production of antibodies. The ill effects of TNFα can also be blocked by etanercept, a synthetic protein which binds to receptors for TNFα and inactivates them. Its combination with methotrexate has been recently shown to be particularly effective in RA, though the combination can seriously lower the body's resistance to bacterial infection. Methotrexate alone is already well-established as a main treatment for RA, despite its potential ill effects.

Attempts have been made to treat severe RA by irradiating all lymphocyte-containing tissues with X-rays, thus destroying the T-cells which are (presumably) doing the damage. Unfortunately improvement was only short-lived.

Other similar conditions: systemic lupus erythematosus

The best-known RA lookalike is 'systemic lupus erythematosus', commonly abbreviated to SLE. The name describes the full-blown skin condition with complications ('systemic' = involving organs and systems apart from, or in addition to, the skin; 'lupus' = wolf, signifying destruction of flesh; 'erythem-' = redness). SLE is a more severe and aggressive inflammatory condition than RA. Vital organs such as the heart, lungs and kidneys may be involved and damaged. In SLE there is also deranged function of the B-lymphocytes, but the antibodies seem to be particularly directed towards the double-stranded DNA of cell nuclei.

Recent work suggests that when body cells die in abnormal ways they may produce sensitising factors which set RA in motion[4]. The recently introduced term 'apoptosis' was derived from Greek: 'apo-' = from; 'ptosis' = falling. The word is used now to describe the planned and programmed death of cells, though it was originally used to refer to the normal shedding of leaves from trees each autumn. When cells are traumatised or infected they may die ('necrosis') with the production of inflammation. When a cell dies at the end of its normal lifespan, or when body structures are being remodelled, a set of complex proteins called 'caspases'[5] brings about a very rapid (20–30 minutes) controlled dissolution of the cell, without the production of inflammation.

In SLE it seems that apoptosis goes wrong and doesn't lead to a quiet and harmless death of cells[6]. Certain chemicals (possibly phosphatidylserine) are left on the surfaces of dying cells. Such cells may then be treated as foreign material by the rest of the body. The consequence seems to be the start of a much more extensive process which damages many tissues other than simply joints, even though in its early stages SLE can produce similar symptoms and signs to RA.

Cause

Proper scientists disdain anecdotes. They are so often misleading. Despite this I shall start with a true story. Its message is difficult to ignore. I had been a regular visiting professor in a Canadian university medical school. My wife and I had used the occasion to take two splendid holidays in a small fishing lodge in Ontario. The owner was a highly athletic man in his early forties who was an expert water-skier. When we first met him he took pride in his skill and seemed to have inexhaustible energy. But when we stayed at the lodge in the following year he was a changed man. He had been struck down quite suddenly, within a week or two, with severe pain in his wrists, knees and ankles, which swelled up. He told us that tests had shown that he had developed severe RA. His athletic activities were greatly curtailed.

This example convinced me that whatever other causes of RA may sometimes operate, some external environmental factor must have set the disease in motion in this man. It is true, of course, that there are inherited diseases of middle age which can appear in people who had previously appeared entirely normal. Huntington's disease is an example. This causes incoordination, progressive dementia and death in middle age. But neither it nor any other disease determined by a single gene defect starts in a middle-aged adult as suddenly as RA did in the case I described.

The possible role of infections

More is known about the cause of a less serious and usually self-limiting disease known as 'reactive arthritis' (previously known as Reiter's disease). This is usually triggered either by a bacterial sexually-transmitted infection, usually with *Chlamydia trachomatis* (which causes discharge from the penis in men) or by a gut infection causing diarrhoea. After a few weeks one or more large joints swell up and become painful. The reaction occurs because a small portion of the protein constituents of an infecting organism, perhaps only a sequence of 10 or 12 amino acids, acts as an antigen and brings about a damaging T-cell defence reaction. Certain genetic variants of the HLA system (see p. 27), especially HLA B27, when triggered by an appropriate infecting organism, may cause 'ankylosing spondylitis', a serious and disabling disease.

Although some environmental factor such as an infection may well be the 'seed' of RA as well as of reactive arthritis, an appropriate genetic inheritance (the 'soil') is also needed. As in reactive arthritis, certain inherited human leucocyte antigens (HLAs) seem to predispose to the disease, though an external trigger is needed to start the disease off. There is a lot of evidence incriminating infections in many varieties of infective-immune disease; but so far no single infectious agent has been identified as the trigger for RA.

'Atopy' describes a common partly inherited allergic constitution, discussed in Chapter 2. It seems to confer some protection against RA, but is associated with asthma. Since atopy describes an individual's strong allergic reaction to external agents, its negative association with RA provides some further evidence in favour of RA being initiated by an infection. Retroviruses (see p. 26) and gut bacteria have been the most intensively studied candidates so far[7]. Parvovirus B19, which causes erythema infectiosum, is common and found worldwide. In children it usually causes a mild and self-limiting disease, though it is sometimes associated with transient joint pains. Most children acquire the infection between the ages of 4 and 10. It appears to be specially associated with juvenile RA. The connection with adult RA is less certain, since antibodies to the virus are found in the majority of adults, but evidence incriminating parvovirus B19 seems to be getting stronger[8].

Many other infections have been suspected of triggering RA (e.g. Lyme disease and flavivirus). Both these infections can be carried by ticks. Sufferers from RA seem to have been more often exposed to cats in the home than those not so exposed, though more data are needed for this association to be convincing.

If an external infecting agent is involved in causing RA, there should often be time and space clustering of cases: i.e. there should be many cases in a particular district, or many cases should occur at around the same time. Such evidence of external infection has been looked for, but not convincingly shown[9]. As far as it goes, this is evidence against a ubiquitous virus infection spread by the air, or by water supplies. However, there is some fascinating historical evidence for an extrinsic triggering infection. Severe RA produces characteristic bone changes. Old skeletons in North America show that RA has occurred there for thousands of years, whereas there is no such evidence from buried bones in Europe until the end of the 15th century. Columbus's sailors returned to Europe in 1493 and are often blamed for the epidemic of syphilis which spread across Europe at that time. It is tempting to suggest that they might have also brought another infection, perhaps parvovirus B19, which might have played some part in RA taking hold in Europe[8]. But this can only be regarded at present as just an intriguing speculation.

I wonder if there might be a parallel with the Epstein-Barr (E-B) virus, which has sometimes been thought to be involved in causing RA. As I have already mentioned in Chapter 3, the E-B virus is a ubiquitous herpes virus which infects most children in Europe and North America. Such children may show no evidence of infection at all, or at worst have a mild respiratory illness or sore throat and think nothing of it. Thereafter they become immune to further infections with the same virus. Those who are unlucky enough not to get infected in childhood, but who acquire infection as adults, may suffer from 'glandular fever' (also known as 'infectious mononucleosis'). In my observation of many cases of this common illness, the symptoms are more severe the older you are when you get it. Glandular fever usually clears up in a few weeks, but it can also occasionally lead to more serious conditions such as Hodgkin's lymphoma.

An analogous scenario could be envisaged for human parvovirus B19. This infects the majority of young children. Is it possible that those unlucky enough to escape childhood infections but who encounter the virus as adults might react adversely and develop RA? If the great majority of adults are already immune to parvovirus B19, time and space clustering of new cases of RA might not necessarily be expected even if the parvovirus was its immediate cause. A large prospective study would be needed to investigate the possibility. It would involve screening young adults for evidence of previous parvovirus B19 infection, to find whether those previously uninfected were those who later developed RA and at the same time developed antibody evidence of parvovirus infection. The possibility is an exciting one, because of the possibilities of opening up more specific therapy than exists at present.

Summary

Rheumatoid arthritis (RA) is a common disabling disease which may affect many joints, but particularly the smaller joints of the hands. Joints are usually affected symmetrically. The joint lining (synovium) is inflamed. Both sections of the body's immune system (both 'B-' and 'T-' lymphocytes) are involved. Damage occurs by release of cytokines such as 'tumour necrosis factor'. The blood often contains autoantibodies known as 'rheumatoid factors'.

Probably the best general statement about the cause of RA is that it is an 'infective-immune' disease. That is, the disease is a response by the body's immune system to a variety of common infective agents, especially viruses. There is probably no inescapable need to regard RA as an 'auto-immune' disease, i.e. one set in motion by the body's immune defences treating one of the parts or organs of the body as if it was foreign. It might rather be that the body's immune defences against an infecting organism may not be specific or targeted accurately enough to attack the invader without harming the individual.

Many viruses and bacteria have at times been linked with RA, though no apparent link has been entirely consistent or stood the test of time. An attractive possibility, not yet disproved, is that an infection of an adult by Epstein-Barr virus, or (more plausibly) parvovirus B19, might initiate rheumatoid changes when someone previously unexposed in childhood first encounters the infection.

9

ALZHEIMER'S DISEASE

Alois Alzheimer (1864–1915), a German psychiatrist, gave a lecture in Tübingen in 1906 describing the case of a 51-year-old woman who had hallucinations with progressively impaired memory and social relationships. He watched her for five years, eventually reporting the post-mortem findings. There were plaques and fibrillary tangles in the brain and arteriosclerotic changes in cerebral blood vessels. Alzheimer said that the condition was a characteristic, peculiar and serious disease of the outer layers of the brain (the cerebral cortex). The disease which Alzheimer described, which now bears his name, has since been recognised as probably the commonest cause of 'senile dementia'. (This term simply means 'lack of mind in old age' but sounds more scientific). Two thirds of people with senile dementia are suffering from Alzheimer's disease (AD), which commonly begins over the age of 65. It is curious that most of what we now know about the disease comes from study of the early-onset type of the disease (which Alzheimer's original patient must have had), even though this makes up only about 10% of all cases.

The typical sufferer first experiences memory disturbances, finding it especially difficult to learn new things and to speak coherently and sensibly. Loss of so-called 'episodic' memory for recent events and episodes is disquieting, but erosion of someone's whole general database of knowledge ('semantic' memory) is devastating. Episodic memory seems to depend particularly on the more central parts of the temporal lobe of the brain, technically the 'amygdala/hippocampus' complex (see Fig.14). The consolidation of memory into a person's knowledge database seems to depend particularly on those parts of the temporal lobes closest to the brain surface. The left side seems more important than the right, at least in right-handed people[*].

---

[*] The localisation of different types of memory has been derived by comparing different diseases or injuries affecting different parts of the brain with the memory disorders which each has been consistently found to produce. Localisation of different functions has also been confirmed by recording the chemical ('metabolic') activity of different parts of the brain while different memory tasks are being attempted and

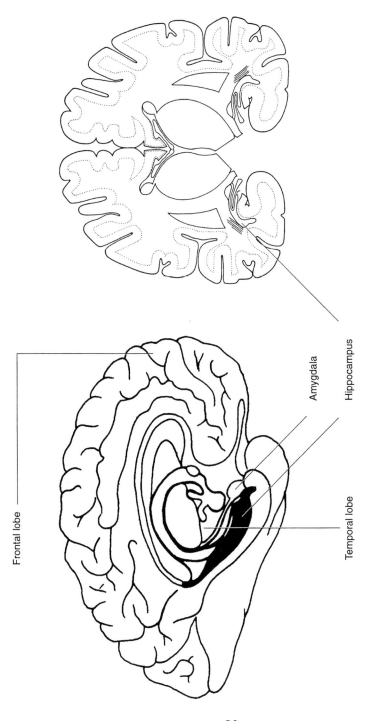

Frontal lobe

Amygdala

Temporal lobe

Hippocampus

Figure 14 On the left is a diagram of the left half of the brain, viewed from the mid-line after removing all the right half of the brain together with the cerebellum and the brain stem. The frontal lobe of the brain lies behind the brow (the frontal bone). The diagram on the right is the brain as it would appear if it was sliced across from top downwards by a 'coronal' section. Both views emphasise the central position of the hippocampus, which makes a curved ridge about 2 inches (5 cm) long, lying in the floor of the lateral ventricle of the brain.

AD seems first to involve the hippocampus complex. This results in loss of memory for recent events. Semantic memory loss follows later when more of the temporal lobe is affected. Imaging techniques consistently show reduced chemical energy provision in the affected areas. Sequential brain scans with magnetic resonance imaging (MRI) show a gradual shrivelling up of those parts of the brain connected with memory, especially the amygdala/hippocampus complex, though later there is more general loss of brain tissue. The fluid-filled ventricles of the brain enlarge and the surrounding brain cortex gets thinner.

With the loss of semantic memory the victim loses his or her personality, has difficulties in recognising people and behaves in an irresponsible and childish manner. Usually five years or so after the mental deterioration of AD has been noticed, the sufferer becomes mute, immobile, rigid, unresponsive and eventually incontinent. Death usually results from accidents or infections, mainly pneumonia. Curiously, the 'sensory-motor cortex', that part of the brain concerned with physical sensation and with the initiation and control of muscle movement, is spared until late in the disease. The sufferer can often still walk about despite being severely demented. The changes of AD develop to different degrees in different parts of the brain, but those parts concerned with higher mental functions like memory and intellectual reasoning are much more affected than those concerned with coordinated muscle movement.

Under the microscope the classic hallmarks of AD are basket-like microscopic tangles inside nerve cells (neurofibrillary tangles) and the building up of flat lumps of structureless starchy material (so-called 'senile plaques'). There is some evidence that plaques appear earlier than tangles. There is also actual loss of brain cells. Tangles are also seen in 'glial' cells (Greek: 'glia' = glue), cells which lie in close apposition to nerve cells. These cells intervene between arteries of blood supply and nerve cell bodies. They presumably convey nutrients across and probably have other functions (see p. 224). Some tangles and even amyloid plaques can be found in brain cells of non-demented elderly people but are much more frequent in AD brains.

different nerve cells activated. This can be done from outside the brain by an imaging technique known as positron-emission tomography(PET). This can quantify local blood flow and also local rate of consumption of glucose by brain cells. In addition, a technique known as 'single photon emission computerised tomography' (SPECT) allows the rates of blood flow in different parts of the brain to be compared. Yet another technique, 'functional magnetic resonance imaging' (fMRI), allows measurement of the local oxygen content of different brain areas.

Metabolic defects

In adults the simple sugar glucose is the brain's main fuel source. Its energy-producing metabolism is impaired in AD. PET scanning shows that there is a reduction in glucose consumption, especially in the hippocampus[1]. The most likely reason for this is that the nerve cells themselves are not working normally and therefore use less glucose. However, it is also possible that a defect in energy supply comes first and that other changes (such as the deposition of neurofibrillary tangles) are actually caused by the energy supply defect. This seems to me rather unlikely because although neurofibrillary tangles are sometimes seen in the brains of people dying from strokes caused by blockage of arteries, they are much less obvious than in AD. But it may be unfair to make a comparison with strokes, which are sudden events. Perhaps slow strangulation of the blood supply to the temporal lobe could yet be the underlying fault in AD, though the progressive relentless involvement of other parts of the brain is difficult to fit with this idea.

A deficiency of the chemical neurotransmitter 'acetylcholine' is characteristic of AD, but is not always found in the same places where glucose consumption rate is reduced. There is also current interest in the finding of reduced concentrations of the excitatory neurotransmitter 'glutamate' (see p. 224) in cortical nerve cells.

Structural changes

It is difficult to distinguish early AD from the normal expected decline in nerve function with age and from other causes of dementia such as furring up of brain arteries (cerebral arteriosclerosis). All the changes in the brain which are characteristic of AD have been seen, to a much smaller degree, in other varieties of dementia. Brain scans show overlap between AD and two other conditions which can be associated with dementia: Parkinson's disease and motor neurone disease (see Chapter 22) – though the microscopical findings in brain cells are different in each of these conditions.

In all three conditions abnormal microscopic particles may be seen inside nerve cells. So-called 'Lewy bodies' are specially characteristic of Parkinson's disease and 'Bunina bodies' of motor neurone disease. Both types of particle contain 'ubiquitin', a protein which when combined with waste proteinaceous material marks it down for later removal. Lewy bodies without any other abnormalities are also found in 'dementia with Lewy bodies', a disease which has yet to find a simpler name. Its symptoms and pathological findings overlap with those of AD, though the outer layers of the brain (the cortex) are mainly affected.

Epidemiology

At the moment there is no completely reliable way to make a positive diagnosis of AD in life except by brain biopsy. This obviously makes it impossible to carry out big population studies. Dementia develops slowly. Lots of elderly people who are not demented have difficulties with memory. So it is difficult to say exactly when a particular individual has developed the disease. What is certain is that AD is very common in the elderly. In the whole population of men and women over 65 the lowest estimate of prevalence of AD I have seen is 1%, but most investigators reckon that it is probably much higher (e.g. 5–10%). By the age of 85 a careful survey has suggested that almost 50% of the population is affected[2] although some authors would regard this as an overestimate. Current estimates are that about 600,000 individuals in the UK are suffering from AD. US President Ronald Reagan and UK Prime Minister Harold Wilson were both said to have suffered from AD, doubtless accounting for their eventual memory loss and failing powers of concentration. Difficulties with memory affect most of us as we get older. But someone like Wilson, who had a phenomenal and celebrated memory, must have found it especially distressing if he realised what was happening to him. This presumably explains Wilson's sudden resignation from the prime ministership.

The cost of AD is not only personal and social: the total annual costs of the disease in the USA have been estimated to approach 70 billion dollars.

Genetic factors

In about 10% of cases AD seems to be genetic and behaves as a dominant inherited characteristic (see p. 60). Some 50 different mutations have already been identified on chromosome 14 for the so-called 'presenilin' gene PS-1, and two on chromosome 1 for the presenilin gene PS-2. Other important genes for AD have been found on chromosomes 21 and 17. In most families with dominant inheritance the disease starts earlier in life than in the sporadic form (e.g. between 35 and 60). The mutations responsible may be connected with the production or function of the amyloid-precursor protein (APP: see below) and with excess production of the 42–43 amino acid fragment Aβ (see below). The list of possible mutations is undoubtedly incomplete.

83

One genetic factor has been definitely linked with late onset sporadic disease. This is the gene responsible for a particular (fat + protein) compound known as apolipoprotein E-epsilon-4 (APOEε4), the genetic code for which is carried on chromosome 19. People with this genetic marker have been known for several years to have a higher than normal risk of developing AD and also an earlier age of onset. People unlucky enough to inherit two copies of the gene (one from each parent) will usually develop AD. It is curious that the gene concerned was first identified as a possible marker for premature atheromatous arterial disease but has proved to have a much closer association with AD.

There also seems to be a link with smoking, which increases the risk of people carrying the APOEε4 gene developing AD. The suggestion has been made that the increased risk which this gene provides is mainly, perhaps exclusively, associated with an infection or recrudescence of infection with *Herpes simplex virus 1* (HSV1), even though neither the particular variety of apolipoprotein, nor HSV1 infection alone, are notably associated in themselves with AD. If this observation is confirmed (and it is currently disputed) finding APOEε4 in the blood will unfortunately not be specific enough to be useful in diagnosing AD. The same applies to the newly-discovered marker gene for AD risk carried on chromosome 12. Another genetic mutation of a neurotransmitter protein (BCHE-K) can apparently multiply the risk of AD thirty-fold.

The genetic instruction code for cells to make amyloid precursor protein lies on chromosome 21. This is the chromosome which is reduplicated in individuals with the well-known common congenital abnormality known as 'Down's syndrome'. It is therefore not unexpected that Down's individuals carrying three copies of chromosome 21, instead of the normal two, have an increased risk of AD, presumably because they make more than normal amounts of amyloid precursor protein.

The multiplicity of genetic risk factors, carried on different chromosomes, make it difficult to envisage a comprehensive unifying hypothesis to account for AD. The difficulties seem to be increasing with each newly-identified risk factor. Almost certainly the disease is not a single entity but rather the end stage of a number of different processes by which brain cells can be damaged.

Cause

It has been said that attempting to understand the cause of AD from the post-mortem brain is like looking out on a battlefield after the war and trying to work out how it all started. However, perhaps we can get some information from the shell cases and other debris left behind. The plaques inside neurones and glial cells have been shown to be composed of a relatively insoluble protein fragment called Aβ amyloid (Greek: 'amylon' = starch). Most animal proteins will slowly dissolve in water. Gelatin is a familiar example of a soluble protein. But other proteins are more like hair or silk. Once formed they cannot easily be broken down or made soluble within the body. Aβ amyloid fragments seem to accumulate particularly in the junctions between individual nerve cells in AD. This seems to be because one of the chemicals which acts as an adhesive (joining adjacent nerve cells together to allow communication between them) is one of the components of amyloid protein. This protein is widespread but found particularly in brain and in platelets (the sticky elements of the blood). It seems that in AD this protein breaks down in an abnormal fashion. Strong evidence for this has come from study of a rare genetic defect in the amyloid precursor protein which causes an affected individual to develop typical AD before the age of 65. A transgenic mouse strain has been developed into which the defective amyloid precursor protein gene has been inserted. The mouse develops in its brain cells plaques, tangles, neuronal degeneration and all the biochemical and pathological abnormalities of AD[3]. Synthetic protein fragments have been identified which can induce the formation of insoluble intracellular deposits similar to those found in AD[4].

The widely-distributed peptide[*] fragment Aβ contains 40 amino acids and does not appear to be damaging. But a larger less soluble fragment, containing 42 amino acids, can be found located at the centre of amyloid plaques. It is tempting to see a similarity between large protein fragments causing damage to neurones through aggregation in AD and the large protein aggregates damaging neurones in Huntington's disease. Huntington's is an inherited condition caused by a mutation which produces abnormal brain proteins. The individual molecules of these proteins are larger than normal because they are extended by a long chain of glutamine residues. Brain cells in Huntington's disease seem unable to break down this abnormal protein, which

---

[*] 'Amino acids' all contain a nitrogen ('amino-') component linked to an acidic chemical group, as the name suggests. DNA contains codes which can instruct the ribosomes in cells to build up peptides and proteins from the 20 different available amino acids. A 'peptide' contains two or more amino acids strung together. The number of amino acids which comprise a 'polypeptide' is undefined, but when the number gets into the high hundreds or thousands a polypeptide is then described as a 'protein'. A small chemical molecule such as the hormone insulin (deficiency of which causes diabetes) can be described either as a large polypeptide or as a small protein.

gradually accumulates in the nuclei of brain cells and destroys them. After a normal childhood and early adult life the victim gets progressive neurological symptoms and dementia. Death occurs inexorably in middle age.

There is a curious point of resemblance between AD and Huntington's disease. In both a polypeptide chain of more than about 40 amino acids is found in the insoluble material: glutamine repeats in the case of Huntington's and the amyloid Aβ components in Alzheimer's. Is it possible that once 40 or more consecutive amino acids have been synthesised by the ribosomes they might turn on themselves, coil up in a ball, trap other amino acids and aggregate into the 'inclusion bodies' which characterise each disease?

Another protein (currently known as AMY117) has been reported to be specially associated with AD plaques, possibly even more closely than Aβ[5]. Proteins sometimes become 'glycosylated', that is, they combine with glucose to form a much less soluble material known as an 'advanced glycation end-product'(AGE). Such modified proteins are not easily broken down within the body. They may even pave the way to a change in structure of amyloid precursor protein[6].

Tau proteins

Analysis of the neurofibrillary tangles in AD has shown them to comprise two kinds of abnormal minute filaments. Most (95%) are paired helical filaments; the remainder are straight. Both are composed mainly of 'tau' protein ('tau' being the English way of writing the Greek letter τ). This is normally produced by nerve cells and found in the microtubules of their axons. In AD the tau proteins contain abnormal quantities of phosphate. They do not bind to microtubules in the normal way, but bind strongly to aluminium. This metal element has been implicated in causing AD, possibly by acting as a co-factor in the formation of neurofibrillary tangles[7].

The picture is at present extremely confusing. Is the excess of phosphate in tau protein caused by an inherited or acquired metabolic fault? The reversible 'phosphorylation' of proteins (the addition of phosphate) regulates virtually all metabolic activities in cells. If the excess phosphate in tau proteins is acquired, is it a primary abnormality or (perhaps) secondary to a non-specific reduction in nerve function resulting in an excess production of adenosine triphosphate (ATP), the source of energy for virtually all chemical processes in the brain and elsewhere? Or is it due to inhibition of a phosphate-removing enzyme (a 'phosphatase')? Many known toxins work by inhibiting phosphatases. This allows one to speculate that a possible cause of AD might be an as yet unrecognised toxin causing excess phosphate attachment to tau proteins.

Animal models

Although gene manipulation has succeeded in creating a convincingly accurate mouse model of AD it has not so far been possible to induce the brain changes of the disease either in mice or rats by injecting ground-up Alzheimer's brain extracts, though primates may be more vulnerable than lower animals. However, it has been reported that extracts of Alzheimer's brains may be toxic to nerve cells living or growing outside the body in tissue culture.

Implications from treatment

Research in AD would be immeasurably helped if there was a blood test by which the diagnosis could be made. Unfortunately there is as yet no such test. A few observations of possible lines of treatment have been made and might shed some light on causation. Some unpublished evidence has suggested that patients with AD have higher than normal concentrations of homocysteine in their blood, suggesting that they might be deficient in the vitamin folate, which assists the metabolism of homocysteine. I doubt whether folate deficiency has much to do with AD. It is inevitable that many demented patients will be eating a folate-deficient diet. If so the elevated homocysteine levels could be a consequence of this. However, it is entirely reasonable to give folic acid supplements to any elderly person who is not also deficient in vitamin B_{12} (even though it probably has nothing to do with AD) because folate deficiency is a recognised cause of neuropsychiatric symptoms. I shall discuss some of the mysteries surrounding folate metabolism further in Chapter 20.

Other associations of Alzheimer's disease

There is current interest in the possibility that 'oestrogens', the collective name for chemicals acting in a specific way as female sex hormones, may give some protection against mental deterioration in AD. If the blood pressure of someone with AD is raised, blood pressure lowering treatment is worthwhile and has been reported to reduce the incidence of dementia in a multi-centre trial. Disease of brain arteries is commonly associated with AD. Since pre-menopausal women may be partly protected against arterial disease by oestrogens, the possible beneficial effects of these drugs may be indirect.

There has been an interesting long-term study of a group of nuns relating linguistic ability in early life, assessed by personal autobiographies written by women in their early twenties, to the development of AD 50–60 years later. Poor linguistic ability was found to be a strong predictor of subsequent development of AD and of poor intellectual function later in life[8]. This observation is difficult to categorise; but complementary results have been reported in another survey[9] in which it was noted that high early educational and occupational attainment may reduce the risk of developing AD later in life. Are these further examples of the physiological generalisation that the more some organ or function is used, the longer it lasts – and vice versa?

There is an important inflammatory element in AD. Many cytokines are activated. Anti-inflammatory drugs such as indomethacin and ibuprofen have a place in treatment. They delay or even inhibit development of AD. All this suggests that an infection may be important as a trigger factor for the disease in susceptible individuals. A virus like HSV1 might act as a trigger. Another pointer to an external pathogenic factor is that there are substantial geographical differences in AD incidence[10]. Unfortunately it is difficult to distinguish AD from other causes of dementia in old age. Victims may live for many years. The disease can only be identified positively in life by brain biopsy. An important series of observations have been made of serial changes in brain size developing over time. If these are plotted graphically, they strongly suggest that AD begins suddenly in the temporal lobe of the brain at a discrete point in time, rather than being a slow progression over decades. It has even been suggested that a spirochaete, a bacterium of the same type that causes syphilis, might be involved as a trigger to set the disease off, though this has not at present been confirmed.

As I have already mentioned, one of the measurable changes in AD is a reduction in concentrations of the neurotransmitter acetylcholine in the brain. Attempts have been made to improve brain function by giving drugs such as tacrine, donepezil, rivastigmine and metrifonate. These drugs inhibit acetylcholine esterase (the enzyme which normally rapidly destroys acetylcholine). They thus increase the amounts of acetylcholine at nerve junctions. In some trials these drugs appear to have brought benefit. Unfortunately this tends to be only short-lasting and is reversed when the drug is withdrawn. Another problem is that these drugs are non-selective and block the action of the enzyme elsewhere, causing a build-up of acetylcholine in places such as the gut, causing nausea and increased gut movements.

There is also recent interest in the neurotransmitter galanin, which appears to stimulate neuronal growth and may play some part in nerve regeneration.

Energy supply to the brain

If AD slowly progresses through the accumulation of some damaging material in brain cells, it would be necessary to invoke some sort of vicious circle to explain why brain damage seems to speed up towards the end. One suggestion has been the 'excitotoxic' theory: that damage of nerve cells by any cause (e.g. impaired blood supply) might liberate excessive amounts of the excitatory neurotransmitters glutamate and aspartate. This would increase metabolic demands on the remaining living nerve cells, release more glutamate and create a vicious circle. I find such ideas difficult to reconcile with evidence that metabolic rate and glucose consumption seem to be especially reduced in those regions of brain most affected by AD.

There is some evidence for specifically maternal inheritance of AD. Surveys have shown that there is a higher than expected ratio of affected mothers to affected fathers among parents of people with the condition. In other words, you are somewhat more likely to develop AD if your mother was affected than if your father was[11]. This points a finger towards mitochondria, the minute energy-supplying structures inside all cells (see p. 225). These are outside cell nuclei and are inherited almost exclusively from the original ovum, i.e. from the mother. Sperms contain very few mitochondria. As mentioned above, affected regions of the brain in AD have a lower metabolic rate and glucose consumption than normal. So perhaps predisposing chromosomal mutations depend on some defect in mitochondrial energy supply to exert their full damaging effect.

Summary

Alzheimer's disease (AD) is probably the commonest cause of loss of mental functions in old age. It affects at least 1% of the population over 65, probably more. There is initial memory loss, but later all intellectual functions are impaired. The brunt of the damage falls on the hippocampal complex, in which energy metabolism is reduced.

There are at least three, possibly more, different dominantly inherited mutations which determine that a person will develop AD. None has yet been linked with the much more common occurrence of sporadic AD. This is marked by brain neurones and glial cells accumulating fibrillary tangles and plaques containing an insoluble starchy material, Aβ amyloid. The larger form of this molecule seems to be less soluble that the smaller form and is particularly associated with AD.

The disease probably starts at a discrete point in time, but the precipitating factors are not known. There have been suggestions that an infection with herpes simplex virus 1 (HSV1) might be the trigger. It seems more likely that the pathological changes diagnostic of AD may be induced by several different routes in people with several different genetic predispositions. In some people with AD the cause seems to lie in their genes; but most cases are sporadic. If AD is triggered by an infection it is particularly difficult to see why sporadic cases should be almost confined to the elderly.

There are many mysteries wrapped up in AD. It is difficult to envisage any single unifying explanation. The epidemiology is extraordinarily difficult. The world awaits a simple but accurate non-traumatic diagnostic test which can be applied prospectively to large populations. Such a test is needed not only for unravelling and making sense of the large number of possible causes, but also for assessing possible treatments and designing trials.

10

PAGET'S DISEASE OF BONE

Sir James Paget was a famous surgeon and teacher at St. Bartholomew's Hospital in London. In 1877 he described a disease of bone known now as 'osteitis deformans' but more often simply as 'Paget's disease'. (One should add 'of bone' since Paget's name is associated with other quite different diseases.) The condition is a curious mix of bone softening and bone overgrowth. It affects most often the lower bones of the spine (the lower lumbar vertebrae and sacrum), the skull and the pelvis, though long bones may also be involved. In about 10% of cases only a single bone or even part of a bone is involved. The disease seldom appears before the age of 40. Thereafter the incidence of new cases steadily increases in frequency. Men are more often affected than women. The first symptom may be pain in the affected bone or bones. If the main lower leg bone (the tibia) is affected, the bone first softens and bends forwards. If the thigh bone (the femur) is involved, it bows outwards. Later the bones thicken and re-ossify in their new shape, which may look 'as though they have been bent by the hands of a giant'. Bones are affected apparently at random and usually asymmetrically, hence the 'deforming' label attached to the disease. One or more bones of the pelvis are commonly involved. The skull is often affected. When men usually wore hats, an early symptom of Paget's disease was the need for a larger size of hat. Bony overgrowth in the skull may compress the auditory nerve on one or both sides, leading to deafness.

The sufferer from extensive Paget's disease has a short, squat figure. The shoulders are bent and the enlarged head hangs forward. The gait is waddling and the sufferer commonly uses a stick. Though muscles are not much affected the bony deformities can make balanced walking difficult (Fig. 15). However, Paget's disease may affect only a single bone (e.g. one vertebral bone in the spine or one lower leg bone). In such cases the diagnosis may be made by accident, perhaps when a routine X-ray is taken. I have seen Paget's disease of the collar bone on one side accidentally revealed in a routine chest X-ray.

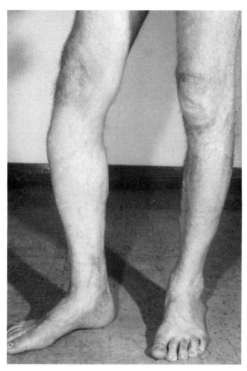

Figure 15 Bowing forwards of the main bone in the right leg (the tibia) in a man with Paget's disease (courtesy of John Kanis).

Under the microscope the bone structure in Paget's disease is grossly disturbed. It has been likened to an irregular mosaic of cement lines. The pattern is due to numerous successive phases of bone absorption and bone regeneration. There is an excess of bone-dissolving cells (osteoclasts) (Greek: 'osteo-' = bone; '-clast' = destruction) but also uncoordinated activity of bone-forming cells (osteoblasts) ('-blast' = bud, germ). Although the affected bones are thickened, enlarged and distorted (Fig. 16), they are porous and not as strong as their gross appearance suggests. Although affected bones very occasionally develop a rare malignant tumour (an osteosarcoma), Paget's disease generally runs a benign course. Lesions develop slowly and the disease seldom shortens life. In unselected post-mortem examinations Paget's disease has been recognised in 3–4% of cases. X-ray population surveys in the USA and Northern Europe suggest a higher prevalence, up to 6% of the adult population.

92

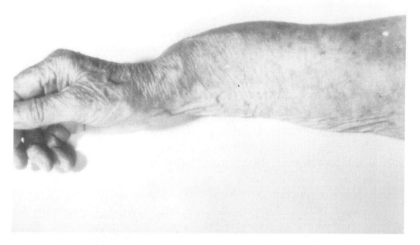

Figure 16A Bowing forwards of the main bone in the lower arm (the radius) in a patient with Paget's disease.

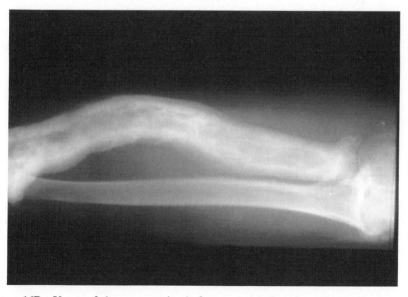

Figure 16B X-ray of the same patient's forearm, showing the coarse enlargement of the radius bone, with increased length and deformity. The adjacent (normal) thin ulnar bone is not affected. In this conventional type of X-ray picture bone appears white and soft tissues and background are black (courtesy of John Kanis).

Cause

The disease is common in Europe, the USA and Australia, but it is uncommon in China, Japan, Scandinavia, the Middle East and Africa. Its prevalence in South America and Mediterranean countries is midway between these. Within the UK the disease is more prevalent in northern than southern parts. All these observations ought to give a clue as to the probable cause. Is this an infection spread in confined spaces? Or is its occurrence favoured by low external temperatures? Most of the commonly involved bones (skull, vertebrae, pelvis and thigh) have a good blood supply, which is increased in Paget's disease. (One clinical sign suggesting the involvement of a bone in Paget's disease is an increase in the temperature of the skin over the bone concerned.)

Most experts at present attribute Paget's disease to a virus infection which gets into bones of a predisposed individual and activates osteoclasts. Electron microscopy of osteoclasts in Paget's disease shows that many have abnormal particles ('inclusion bodies') inside cells, or even inside the cell nuclei. These are not found in normal osteoclasts, but might be viral or bacterial products. Possible viruses include the paramyxoviridae, especially measles (MV), respiratory syncytial virus (RSV) and canine distemper virus (CDV). Simian virus 5 and parainfluenza virus type 3 have also been implicated. Various identifiable portions of viruses (e.g. antigens of MV and RSV) have been demonstrated in osteoclast inclusions. So is the problem solved? I think not.

There are difficulties in accepting the virus hypothesis. The virus components and inclusion bodies in osteoclasts certainly suggest that viruses could be the cause of Paget's disease. But they might just be opportunistic travellers. A recent reviewer pointed out[1]: (1) that there is little evidence of different blood concentrations of antibodies to MV, RSV, CDV or parainfluenza viruses when Paget patients are compared with normal subjects; (2) not all osteoclasts in Paget's disease contain the (presumed) viral inclusions; (3) similar inclusions have been observed in some rare conditions (e.g. non-pagetic giant cell tumours, osteopetrosis, pycnodysostosis and familial expansile osteolysis): thus the inclusions would have to alter osteoclast function differently in non-Paget disorders; (5) no infectious agent has yet been extracted from pagetic tissue; (6) the paramyxoviridae are ubiquitous whereas there are striking geographical differences in Paget's prevalence.

Paget's disease seems to be unique to man. Why is this? Postmortem and radiological surveys from Europe estimate a 3% prevalence for the population over 40 and 5% for the population over 55. It is extraordinary that there is no animal model for such a common human disorder. Paget's is a disease of the elderly: perhaps animals don't live long enough to get it? Is there some exclusively human habit of diet, posture or social behaviour which predisposes to the disease? The enormous variations in prevalence in different parts of the world and different ethnic groups point to an environmental cause. People in Europe, North America and Australasia are more affected than those in the Third World. Paget's disease often runs in families, but truly genetic influences are not strong[1]. Only five examples of Paget's disease in identical twins have been recorded. It is almost impossible to rule out the influence of shared family environments such as diet in causing familial aggregation of cases.

Why should the disease pick out certain bones preferentially (e.g. the long leg bones, pelvis, spine and skull)? It is said that the right side of the body is more often affected than the left. If so, why? Since bone destruction seems to start Paget's disease off, it seems relevant to ask what external agents might start off bone weakening by stimulating the osteoclasts, the specialised cells which actively dissolve or destroy bone.

Osteoclast stimulation by bacteria

Suppose viruses are irrelevant. Suppose they are simply picked up by pagetic osteoclasts and do not make those cells grow larger and more active. Is there any other extrinsic source of material known to stimulate osteoclasts strongly and which could enter bone via the blood-stream? (The natural history of Paget's disease seems best explained by the initiating agent arriving in the blood and settling at random in bones.) Many well-known bacteria have the ability to destroy bone, though bone abscesses (collections of pus) are not seen in Paget's disease. But many less virulent non-oxygen requiring ('anaerobic') bacteria can destroy bone. In particular, a bacterium called *Actinobacillus actinomycetemcomitans* (AA) has potent bone-resorbing activity. It causes local infection of tooth sockets (periodontitis) especially in children[2]. Antibodies to this organism and to many other mouth bacteria can be detected in the blood of people with periodontitis[3]. The antibodies produced may have a protective role.

Since circulating antibodies to several anaerobic mouth bacteria can often be found in normal people, the organisms responsible must presumably get into the bloodstream. I have speculated[4] that AA (for example) might get into bone and lodge there, perhaps in thick bone tissue in which oxygen tension might be relatively low. The frequency

95

of involvement of long bones is proportional to their volume. If AA bacteria get into bone and are taken into osteoclasts – which share most properties of phagocytes (scavenger cells) and probably derive from a common precursor – they would not be expected to cause inflammation.

Bacteria were looked for in affected bones in Paget's disease nearly a century ago and intermittently since, without success. But AA is a small fastidious non-motile bacillus (a particular type of bacterium) which is slow-growing and difficult to study. It might persist only in a single small focus within each affected bone and might have been overlooked. For example, *Tropheryma whippelii* (causing Whipple's disease, a serious condition initially affecting the intestinal wall) and *Helicobacter pylori* (causing peptic ulcers) were overlooked for decades. AA bacteria can grow and even multiply inside cultured human cells[5]. If symbiosis (Greek: 'living together') between AA bacteria and osteoclasts became established within bone, the infected osteoclasts might be spared immunological destruction, as are human cells infected by *Tropheryma whippelii*.

When growing in test-tube cultures outside the body AA bacteria produce several powerful osteoclast-stimulating materials. Some of these can be readily washed off the surface of AA bacteria in culture. Thus it is possible that material from a small focus of AA infection could diffuse within bone, stimulating and changing osteoclast function in the surrounding region. The rate of progression of Paget's disease can be followed by serial X-rays. From its origin in a long bone the disease process only moves along very slowly, at a rate of between ¼ to ¾ inch per year[6] (see Fig. 17). Such a slow rate of progression would be entirely compatible with the very slow diffusion of large osteoclast-stimulating molecules through bone matrix (see Table opposite).

An advancing front of Paget's disease created by the very slow diffusion of large protein molecules seems to me a more credible explanation than the advance of an incredibly slow infection down a long bone. The way in which the advance of Paget's disease may peter out half way along the length of a long bone also suggests the progressive weakening of a chemical osteoclastic stimulus.

Knowing the rate of progression of Paget's disease changes in a long bone it is possible to work out roughly when the disease began in that bone. The data 'suggest that Paget's disease may be a disease of teenagers and young adults'[6] but one which can take many years before it causes symptoms or gross deformities.

Humans with severe periodontitis have increased circulating antibodies to AA bacteria. Simple brushing of the teeth is well-known to

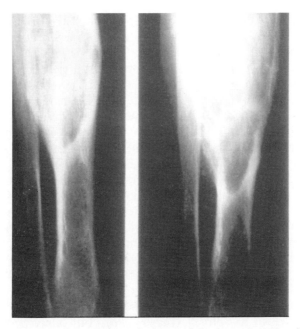

Figure 17 Two X-rays of the same main bone of the lower leg (the tibia), taken at different stages of the disease. The knee joint (not shown) lies above the upper part of the X-rays, and the ankle joint (also not visible) lies below the lower part of the X-rays. The upper part of the tibia is swollen and distorted by Paget's disease. Half-way down the bone a V-shaped line of demarcation separates active disease above, where the bone density is diminished, and normal bone below. The X-ray on the right was taken 3 years after that on the left. It shows how very slowly the disease progresses. The advancing front of disease has moved only about one inch down the leg (X-rays by courtesy of John Kanis).

Table of typical molecular diffusion rates

Times for 50% of molecules to move by diffusion alone

Distance	Glucose	Small protein
1 micron (1/1000mm)	1/1000 second	1/100 second
10 microns (1/100mm)	1/10 second	1 second
1mm	16 minutes	4 hours
1cm	26 hours	17 days
10cm	4 months	5 years

send bacteria into the bloodstream. Scaling and root planing in people with periodontitis has been observed to increase AA antibody concentrations over a 6–12 month period. Is it possible that conservative dentistry, in which people in developed countries take pride, might sometimes spread AA and other potential osteoclast-stimulating organisms from the mouth into the bloodstream and thence into bones? This hypothesis could be tested by examining old embedded pagetic bone sections by the modern technique of immunocytochemistry. If marker antigens of AA or of other pathogenic oral bacteria were found in or close to osteoclasts, or if antibodies to one or more of them were found in high titre in Paget's disease, further investigation of the possible role of bacterial infection would be worthwhile. Unfortunately I have not yet located an academic department of pathology which holds a stock of old embedded sections of Paget's diseased bones and which has sufficient interest to make a pilot study.

My clinical impression is that gross deformities of the Paget's disease type have become much rarer than they were when I was first a medical student. If my hypothesis is correct, this could be due not only to current treatment of Paget patients with biphosphonates, which induce osteoclast apoptosis (see p. 75), but also perhaps to the widespread use of broad-spectrum antibiotics to which all mouth anaerobic bacteria are to some extent sensitive.

There are few epidemiological data about dental problems in Paget patients, though dentists often make the initial diagnosis. In any case, distal bone foci are probably established years before the disease starts to produce symptoms and signs. Recently a questionnaire about complications was answered by 292 randomly selected Paget's disease patients. They rated the state of their mouth and teeth as unhealthier than that of matched controls. Paget's patients more often reported pain on opening the mouth[7]. The very rare condition of juvenile Paget's disease (idiopathic hyperphosphatasia) is associated with premature loss of teeth.

Invoking mouth bacteria as the cause of Paget's disease helps to account for the unique affliction of man. Most animals' teeth are widely-spaced and a roughage diet is protective. Only sheep have periodontitis comparable to ours. AA antibodies have been reported in diseased sheep, though other species of mouth bacteria predominate. Sheep have been kept for up to 15 years as pets or for antibody production. They sometimes even need false teeth, so it might be worth looking out for Paget lesions in elderly sheep with bad teeth. I have spoken to vets about this, but so far have drawn a blank. This is probably because my hypothesis is wrong; but it would be amusing if it proved to be correct.

Jokes are unfortunately rare in science. In his 1969 monograph on

Paget's disease[8] Hugh Barry wrote: 'One feels that when the secret is given up it may be so obvious that it is right there under our noses'. It would be ironic if the cause of Paget's disease eventually proved to lie exactly there!

Summary

Paget's disease of bone is a deforming condition affecting mainly large bones in a random fashion. There is first stimulation and proliferation of bone-destroying cells (osteoclasts). These cause bone softening, usually with bending and distortion. Later bone-forming cells (osteoblasts) take over and proliferate. New bone is laid down, often leaving bizarrely deformed long bones and a curious mosaic pattern when bone sections are examined under the microscope.

Under the microscope Pagetic osteoclasts usually contain foreign particles, some of which might be viruses. However, the viruses apparently associated with these osteoclasts could be opportunistic rather than causative. Some mouth bacteria can destroy bone. One (*Actinobacillus actinomycetemcomitans*) can grow and even multiply inside human cell lines in culture, producing potent osteoclast-stimulating materials. An (as yet) untested hypothesis is that a small focus in a bone of this bacterium, or of one of the other periodontitis-causing bacteria, might gradually spread its chemical influence to activate osteoclasts, the first stage in Paget's disease. The focus in each bone might be small and easily overlooked, as other intracellular bacteria have been in the past.

11

ENDOMETRIOSIS

Endometriosis (EMT) is a bizarre condition. It describes a situation in women in which the normal inner lining of the womb (uterus) is not confined to its normal situation. It has appeared in one or more places outside the womb, usually within the abdominal cavity and most often on the surface of the ovaries. During the reproductive years, some of this inner lining (the 'endometrium') is shed each month, with consequent bleeding (the 'period'). The menstrual cycle is indirectly (via the ovary) controlled by circulating chemical substances (hormones) which are secreted into the bloodstream from the pituitary gland, lying deep inside the skull at the base of the brain. The ovarian hormones act on chemical receptors in the endometrium telling it to shed its old lining cells and regrow its lining at the end of each month, unless other chemical instructions have been given to the womb by secretions from a newly-fertilised egg (ovum).

Unfortunately these effects can be as true for endometrium outside the womb as for the normal endometrium lining the womb. Therefore a lump of endometrial tissue which has somehow got into the abdominal cavity – perhaps stuck on to a piece of the gut – may shed cells and perhaps bleed slightly each month. This can cause abdominal pain at the time of a woman's period by irritating the smooth lining of the abdominal cavity (the 'peritoneum'). If the blood does not leak out it may be retained in the endometrial tissue itself, forming dark-coloured ('chocolate') cysts.

The cause of the pain is rather similar to the pain which some women get in between periods, the well-known 'mittelschmerz' ('middle-pain'). This is produced by slight irritation of the peritoneum when a new egg breaks out of an ovary and briefly enters the peritoneal cavity on its way to one of the two fallopian tubes, which convey it to the womb. If it has been fertilised it becomes implanted in the endometrium about nine days later.

EMT is extremely common in developed countries. In the USA it has been reported in about 70% of adolescent girls complaining of chronic pelvic pain. EMT severe enough to cause symptoms affects between 3% and 7% of all women between the ages of 20 and 45 in developed countries, but in much lesser degree it has been recognised in most women at some stage of their reproductive years. Overall prevalence in the general female population has been estimated as 10%. Prevalence increases with age in pre-menopausal women. It is also associated with shorter (and therefore more frequent) menstrual cycles.

The prevalence of EMT in undeveloped countries has never been reliably evaluated. African women are generally believed to be relatively unaffected. This seems to be borne out by the paucity of case reports from Central Africa. I have been able to find only one such report published in the last 30 years[1]. It might be relevant that the five women reported in this paper were professionals: two were nurses, one a pharmacist, one a school teacher and one a secretary – i.e. all were highly educated. I could find no published survey of naturally-occurring abdominal EMT in Indian women. In terms of publications about EMT during the last 30 years, there have been 1200 from the USA, about 250 from the UK, none from Saudi Arabia and only the one (already mentioned) from Central Africa. Either the condition is very rare in these parts of the world, or doctors there do not report it in medical journals.

There is some evidence of genetically-determined susceptibility to EMT, but no clearly defined Mendelian (see p. 134) pattern of inheritance. When disease is extensive it is associated with infertility. It is sometimes said to be a cause of infertility but it is much more likely that infertility and EMT share a common cause. Treating or removing EMT lesions does not usually restore fertility, though a recent report has been more encouraging.

Although the pain of EMT occurs particularly at the same time as menstruation, for obvious reasons, it is also a cause of vague and ill-defined abdominal pain. Diagnosis can only be made for sure by inspecting the peritoneal surface. This can obviously be done when the abdomen is opened surgically, but it can also be done, though with greater difficulty, by the use of a laparoscope (an illuminated hollow tube which is inserted into the abdomen via a small incision). The lesions appear as superficial bluish-red patches or as 'chocolate cysts' containing old changed blood. They most commonly occur on the surface of the ovaries but can be found anywhere in the abdominal cavity: on the pelvic organs, on the inner abdominal wall, on the surface of some parts of the gut, or on the surface of the liver. Patches may also be seen in unusual places, difficult to inspect, such as the lower surface of the muscular diaphragm, which separates the chest from the abdominal cavity. Sometimes actual lumps of endometrial tissue may resemble, and be mistaken for, a tumour mass. Occasionally lesions can occur within the abdominal wall, or even outside the abdominal cavity altogether.

Under the microscope tissue in the EMT patches resembles normal endometrium, but some differences have been noted when the tissue is cultured in the laboratory. It produces two proteins which are not produced when normal uterine endothelium is cultured. In addition, it fails to produce three other proteins which normal endometrial cells produce. We do not know whether these results indicate a true difference in endometrial cells themselves, or whether their synthetic capabilities have been altered by the unusual environment.

One obvious and generally accepted line of treatment is to interfere with the hormones which control the menstrual cycle and endometrial bleeding, though inevitably this impairs fertility. Removal of the ovaries usually produces complete cure and relief of symptoms. The preferred conservative treatment of severe cases in many centres is careful and accurate destruction of the aberrant endometrial tissue. This can conveniently be done with a laser light beam, either at open operation or via a laparoscope (see above). Active lesions absorb light energy on their dark surfaces. The controlled light beam does not penetrate deeply enough to damage the normal organ below. Laser treatment of the lesions themselves is effective in relieving pain, even though it does not usually improve fertility.

Cause

Current theories to explain endometriosis

The simplest explanation (the 'transplantation theory') is that one or more of the small lumps of endometrium which are shed each month from the lining of the uterus find their way through (up) a fallopian tube into the abdominal cavity. This idea, best described as the 'retrograde menstruation' hypothesis, was first put forward by John Sampson in the 1920s. It is supported by the frequency with which EMT deposits are found on the surface of the ovaries.

Fig. 18 illustrates the relationship between the abdominal cavity (lined by the smooth peritoneum), the two ovaries, the two fallopian tubes, the uterus, and the vagina. The normal function of the fallopian tubes is to convey an egg, newly-liberated from an ovary, from the peritoneal cavity to the inside of the womb. The complicated arrangement normally gives good protection against infection from outside the body getting into the abdominal cavity. The neck of the womb (Latin: 'cervix' = neck) is normally closed, though it opens to let out

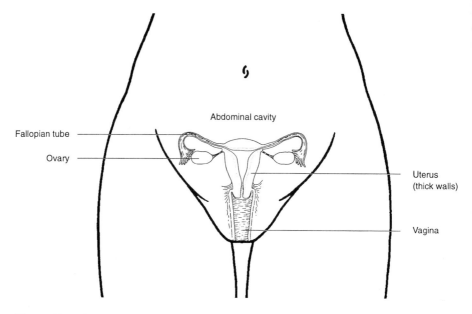

Figure 18 Diagram of the spatial disposition of the internal female organs of reproduction.

the menstrual blood and shed endometrium once a month. It is also negotiable by male sperms deposited in the vagina. They can swim upstream, like miniature tadpoles[*], into the cavity of the uterus. If they encounter an egg in a fallopian tube, or possibly in the uterus itself, it can be fertilised. The cavity of the uterus connects with the abdominal (peritoneal) cavity via the two uterine (fallopian) tubes (see Fig. 18) which end closely applied to the two ovaries. Each tube is about 4 inches (10cm) long. The opening of the tubes into the uterus is very small, the thickness of a bristle. The complex anatomy seems to have evolved to provide the maximum protection against infection getting from the uterus up into the fallopian tubes, which can cause 'salpingitis', and up into the peritoneal cavity, causing 'peritonitis'.

According to the transplantation theory, the probability of a woman developing EMT can be regarded as quantitative and dependent on the interplay of various factors:

1 large amounts of endometrial tissue somehow getting into the abdominal cavity;

[*] 'Polywogs' in the USA.

2 the inherent ability of tissues in the pelvis to support transplantation;

3 a combination of (1) and (2).

Other possibilities have been considered. One is that the lining membrane of the abdominal cavity (the 'mesothelium') changes its character and forms typical endometrium-like glands and tissue. This situation is described as 'c(o)elomic metaplasia'. Another suggestion is that the lining of the womb is not itself transplanted but that chemicals are produced by endometrial tissue which make tissues in other places turn into endometrium. Perhaps the body's immunological defence system somehow encourages abnormal sites of endometrial growth.

Retrograde menstruation

It seems to me, as it has seemed to many others[2] that the Sampson theory of implantation of menstrual endometrium is by far the best explanation of EMT. The suggestion has been made that retrograde menstruation is common, perhaps nearly a universal occurrence. This implies that instead of all the endometrial lining tissue shed each month passing out through the cervix into the vagina, some gets back through the fallopian tubes into the peritoneal cavity, perhaps helped by muscular contractions of the uterus. Living endometrial cells have been identified in fluid in the abdominal cavity in about 50% of all pre-menopausal women[3].

Previous pelvic infection makes EMT more likely and more severe, presumably because of obstructed passage of menstrual material through the cervix. Could the use of tampons by women in industrialised countries be a cause of retrograde menstruation and hence predispose to EMT? Although tampons are loose-fitting, might they partially obstruct free menstrual flow? A survey by the American Endometriosis Association showed that rates of tampon use by women with EMT were similar to those of the population not using tampons, though women with EMT had started to use tampons earlier than those without the disease. In a small survey of tampon use, comparing 100 users with a similar number of non-users, long-term tampon users (14 years or more) were 3.6 times more likely to have EMT than non-users. The 'confidence intervals' for this ratio were wide (1.05 to 13.5)[4]. So tampon use probably has a small effect in encouraging EMT, though it cannot be a major factor. The subject would clearly repay further epidemiological research.

A great mystery which needs explaining is why EMT is not much more common than it is, hence the current interest in a possible immunological cause (e.g. deficient 'T-cell' lymphocyte function: see p. 26). This theory supposes that the peritoneal lining membrane which surrounds the abdominal organs is immunologically protected against bits of endometrium grafting themselves onto some part of the abdominal organs or onto the peritoneal lining membrane. Various rather unimpressive differences in immune function have been reported between women with EMT and women without. But the obvious way to test this theory is to look for the same condition in animals.

Endometriosis in animals

Rodents lack a menstrual cycle and don't get spontaneous EMT. Rabbits lack the so-called 'luteal' phase of the human cycle. Thus animal research on EMT has only proved feasible in primates. The closest animal model of the human disease is that in baboons, which have a 33-day menstrual cycle which continues throughout the year, even in captivity. In a survey of baboons examined under anaesthesia only 4 out of 52 (8%) previously unoperated baboons of proven fertility had a few small plaques of endometrial tissue in the abdominal cavity, outside the uterus. The lesions were mostly small white plaques with pigmented spots, unlike the appearance of human EMT lesions, though occasional typical blue/black cysts were seen. Furthermore, baboon EMT was not seen on the surface of the ovary, where it is commonest in women. Surgical opening of the abdominal cavity in baboons leads later to a great increase in the number and extent of EMT lesions[5]. Rather similar though more limited observations have been made in other primates. EMT has been produced consistently, though to a variable extent, by placing lumps of endometrial tissue into the abdominal cavity of cynomolgous monkeys. The consequent reduction in fertility was related to the extent of EMT. 'Spontaneous' EMT has been reported in rhesus monkeys, most of whom had been exposed to surgical operations. EMT can be induced in female rhesus monkeys whose immune system has been damaged by long-term dioxin exposure. Since this toxin affects ovarian function it may alter oestrogen levels, which could be important.

Requirements for autografting of endometrium

For the tissue to establish itself in the abnormal situation certain key steps are required: the new tissue needs to adhere to the basement membranes of cells of the host tissue; local dissolution of protein has to clear a path for growth; the endometrial tissue cells need to migrate into the colonised host tissue; the grafted tissue needs to acquire new blood vessels if it is to get larger than one or two millimetres in diameter. Despite these difficulties, most experimental work suggests that lumps of endometrium are easily able to survive and grow outside the womb.

Partial obstruction of the cervix is associated with EMT. Previous pelvic infections, leading to fibrous adhesions keeping the fallopian tubes open rather than flat shut, are also a risk factor. If the non-pregnant uterus contracts and raises its internal pressure the conditions for retrograde (reversed) flow could exist, but only if the uterine/fallopian tube junction does not contract at the same time. My guess is that the entry of individual endometrial cells into the peritoneal cavity is harmless. But if a small lump of endometrial tissue (not just a single cell or two) gets into the peritoneal cavity the tissue could stick onto the peritoneal lining membrane and grow. A lesion of EMT would have appeared.

The animal results seem to me to speak rather powerfully against any immunological theory. If bits of endometrium can easily be induced to stick onto and grow on abdominal organs in normal non-human primates whose female pelvic anatomy closely resembles human female anatomy, why don't all women get EMT if retrograde menstruation is as common as most people say it is?

Pressures in the female reproductive organs

A particular interest of mine has always been pressures in blood vessels (see Chapters 15 and 16). It is thus natural for me to see the uterus as having two valves in series: the cervix and the junction between uterine cavity and fallopian tube. A rise of pressure in the abdominal cavity (e.g. from straining at stool) will preferentially close off the thin fallopian tubes, because the thick-walled uterus will more strongly resist collapse by external pressure. Any material in the tubes will therefore be forced in towards the uterine cavity. But when abdominal pressure falls again, the pressure in the cavity of the uterus will be briefly higher than that in the abdomen, so that any unattached contents will tend to move up the fallopian tubes and into the abdominal cavity. In particular, if the intra-abdominal pressure has been raised for many hours (rather than just for a minute during straining at stool) the pressure inside the cavity of the womb would be expected to be about the same as that in the abdominal cavity.

I envisage the following scenario, illustrated diagrammatically in Fig. 19. The normal situation is shown in A, in which there is a uniformly distributed low pressure of about 5 mmHg above the

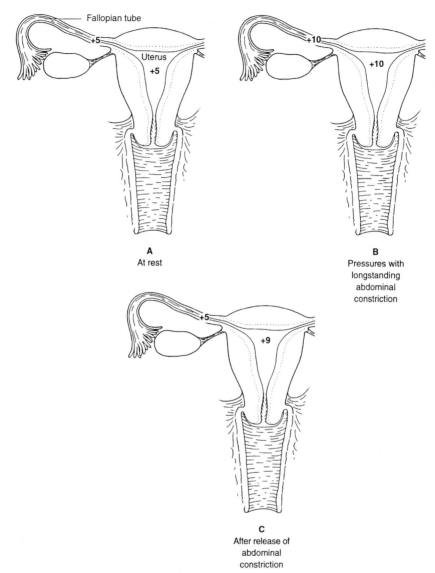

Figure 19 Gross anatomy of uterus and fallopian tubes indicating the probable relative pressures (in mmHg) at different sites. The normal situation is shown in A. B shows the situation which would be expected during the application of a tight constricting abdominal garment, during which all intra-abdominal pressures are increased to the same extent. C shows the hypothetical but plausible relative pressures immediately after removing the constricting garment (see text). Unless the thick muscular uterine wall relaxes completely, the intra-uterine pressure will not fall back to its normal level until some uterine contents have been extruded either through the cervix or up the fallopian tubes.

surrounding atmospheric pressure. During longstanding abdominal constriction all these pressures would be increased, as at B. Immediately after taking off a constricting abdominal garment the pressure within the thick-walled uterus would not be expected to fall back to normal until some of the uterine contents had been expelled. This might lead to a situation such as in C, in which there might then be a substantial and prolonged pressure gradient favouring movement of uterine contents up the fallopian tubes and towards the peritoneal cavity.

This line of reasoning makes me hazard a guess that what garments a women wears while she is menstruating could be important. In particular if the garments produce a sustained rise of intra-abdominal pressure by being tight-fitting, I suspect that retrograde menstruation might occur when the garments are taken off. I also suspect that non-human primates have little propensity to EMT because they do not wear constricting garments. Could the almost universal wearing of sarees by Indian women protect them against EMT? I assume that they have no necessity for, and do not wear, tight, constricting abdominal garments.

I conducted a computerised 'Medline' medical literature search over the last 30+ years for 'endometriosis' to see how many of the more than 5000 references mentioned 'India' or 'Indian' in the context of spontaneous EMT. The answer was only one, as an aside in an article about septicaemia. I have already mentioned the single report from central Africa. I have also found no reports of EMT from Saudi Arabia, in which country all women wear loose-fitting chadors (black enveloping garments). It seems clear that no research doctor working in India, central Africa or Saudi Arabia has much interest or experience in EMT, which would be compatible with my hypothesis. I have not been able to find any epidemiological evidence about garment wearing and EMT. But I would predict that EMT should be rare in places where women do not wear garments which increase intra-abdominal pressure.

If I had all possible facilities to investigate the cause of EMT I should try to devise means for measuring all the pressures at different points in the system. Perhaps those who maintained a high pressure in their abdominal cavity might be relatively protected until the intra-abdominal pressure was suddenly reduced (e.g. when someone takes a constricting garment off). At this moment a previously high pressure surrounding both uterus and fallopian tubes would fall; but there would be a finite time gap during which the pressure inside the uterine cavity would exceed the pressure surrounding the fallopian tubes, because the rigid thick-walled uterus would not immediately relax.

This would set the stage for movement of uterine contents up the fallopian tubes. This is of course pure speculation, but hydrodynamically it is plausible[6].

At least one other pressure-dependent cause of retrograde menstruation can be envisaged. During the first 3 days of the menstrual cycle contractions normally start at the top (fundus) of the uterus and move down towards the cervix. But pinching or even touching of the cervix has been obvserved sometimes to reverse the pattern of intra-uterine pressure changes in menstruating women[7]. This suggests yet another pressure-related hypothesis for endometriosis: that such contractions might be induced by intercourse and encourage retrograde menstruation. Could any of the puzzling geographical distribution of endometriosis be culturally determined? Intercourse during menstruation is expressly forbidden by many religions (e.g. Ezekiel 18, v.6).

Intra-abdominal interstitial fluid pressure

The kind of pressure I have been discussing is easy to understand: the simple hydrostatic or solid tissue pressure exerted when the heart contracts, when an artery constricts, or when the uterus at term expels its fetus. However, there exists a space between tissue cells which contains a small amount of so-called 'interstitial' fluid. Amazingly, the pressure in that fluid is normally subatmospheric, about -7 mmHg, or about -1 inch of water pressure[*].

Our body is being gently squeezed together by the pressure of the atmosphere above us. Dropsy (oedema) arises when the pressure in tissue fluid rises above the atmospheric pressure, thus allowing tissues to be separated by retained fluid. The fluid in the abdominal cavity is on average also held at a similar subatmospheric pressure. So there will normally always be a small pressure gradient tending to move free fluid from the vagina into the uterus and from the uterus into the peritoneal cavity. The pressures concerned are very small, but will be continually present. Whether they have any relevance at all to EMT will need some difficult measurements to determine.

---

[*] The reasons for this are complicated and difficult to explain briefly. The negative interstitial pressure is generated by the 'osmotic' pressure exerted by the proteins in the blood plasma, tending to suck fluid out of the interstitial space and into the blood stream.

Summary

Endometriosis (EMT) is a common condition in which small portions of bluish-red tissue which appear to have come from the inner lining of the womb (the endometrium) are found on the surface of various internal organs, predominantly those in the abdominal cavity, especially the ovary. Similar lesions can much less commonly appear in other places. EMT can cause chronic pain, especially pelvic pain, particularly at the time of the 'period'. It is associated with reduced fertility. Although other explanations have been offered, the likeliest seems to be that the cause is retrograde menstruation, that is, that some of the shed womb lining gets up into the abdominal (peritoneal) cavity and sticks on some organ or lining surface. The process may be facilitated by some immunological process, but this may not be an essential factor. Pressure changes at different parts of the pelvic organs are probably of greater importance. One suggestion – never previously made or published as far as I am aware – is that the clothing worn by menstruating women might be relevant. In addition, sexual intercourse during menstruation could also, in theory at least, encourage retrograde movement of uterine contents.

12

CHRONIC FATIGUE SYNDROME – so-called 'ME'

Every general physician (internist) or general practitioner has been consulted by people with chronic fatigue syndrome (CFS). Unfortunately most patients with this condition prefer to describe themselves as having 'myalgic encephalomyelitis' or 'ME'. This description is inaccurate. It sounds impressive but it annoys doctors a lot. The widespread use of the term is one of the reasons why patients often get a raw deal from the medical profession. Doctors resent having to accept a spurious and inaccurate self-diagnosis. Although the condition can often be correctly described as 'myalgic' (Greek: 'my-' = muscle; 'algi-' = pain), there is no evidence whatsoever for active inflammation in the brain and spinal cord (Greek: 'en-' = in; kephal-' = head; 'myel-' = marrow: i.e. spinal cord; adjectival suffix '-itis' = 'inflammation of').

As it is currently defined, CFS implies that for at least six months there has been persistent or relapsing fatigue which does not resolve with bed rest and which is severe enough to reduce average daily activity by at least 50%. Other chronic conditions including previous psychiatric disease must have been excluded. There may also be a gradual onset of symptoms, mild fever or chills, sore throat, tender lymph glands, muscle weakness with pain or discomfort, excessively lengthy post-exercise fatigue, headaches, flitting joint pains, sleep disturbances and minor psychological symptoms. In the last century such a condition was described as 'neurasthenia' (Greek: 'asthenes' = weak). 'Weak nerves' is not a bad description of CFS. I shall argue that the fault probably lies in the brain rather than in muscles or glands.

Applying strict criteria for the diagnosis of CFS excludes all but a few percent of people complaining of long-standing fatigue. In most cases of CFS there has been no well-defined or consistent abnormality either on clinical examination or laboratory investigation.

Epidemiology

Although some apparent epidemics of CFS have been reported since their first description in 1934 there have been few such reports

113

recently. Cases nowadays are almost invariably sporadic. In different series, mean age has been around 33. About twice as many women as men have been victims. Professional workers may be overrepresented. The prevalence in different surveys in developed countries has been about 50 cases per 100,000 population, though with very strict diagnostic criteria prevalence has been as low as 5 per 100,000.

Cause

Most authors suspend judgement about a possible cause of CFS. In scientific journals about two thirds of authors reject tangible 'organic' (i.e. non-psychological) causes for the condition. By contrast about two thirds of authors writing in national newspapers and women's magazines favour organic causes. The easy approach is to say that organic and psychological factors are inextricably linked. This may be true but is none the less a useless hypothesis because it is untestable.

Since short-lasting fatigue follows many different virus infections is CFS simply a non-specific response to several possible triggers? Many viruses have been suggested as causes of CFS (e.g. Coxsackie B, human herpesvirus-6 and Epstein-Barr virus, the latter well known as the cause of glandular fever). All are common. Evidence of previous infection by one of these viruses can often be found in normal people. Anti-viral agents have not so far helped in treatment. However, a recent report from Australia provided good evidence of a causal relation between a single exposure to the infecting organism *Coxiella burneti* and the later development of CFS[1]. This organism is a very small bacterium (technically one of the 'rickettsiae') which is endemic in some cows and ewes and infects people who inhale the organisms in an aerosol. There is also fairly strong evidence that CFS more often follows glandular fever than other febrile conditions[2].

Are CFS patients genetically predisposed to react adversely and excessively to a virus or other infective trigger? Have CFS patients a psychological make-up which renders them specially liable to develop CFS after a minor illness which leaves most people unscathed? If so, is this vulnerable psychological predisposition itself genetically determined? The case remains open. There is some evidence of altered immunological mechanisms in CFS, but it is maddeningly inconsistent. CFS has been regarded as a non-specific complex of symptoms related to various causal agents able to induce an immune response. Such a hypothesis is imprecise. It cannot be rigorously tested.

Could CFS be due to the accidental ingestion of a poison? For example, an illness known as ciguatera is caused by eating extremely

114

poisonous chemicals called ciguatoxins, which are found in certain Oriental and Caribbean fish. Some of these fish are highly prized culinary delicacies but need careful preparation to remove the poisonous parts. The toxin damages 'ion channels', structures in cell membranes which are exquisitely sensitive to various external triggers. Ciguatoxins can damage these structures semi-permanently leading to a chronic condition which is virtually identical to CFS[3]. There is extreme fatiguability and often muscle and joint pains. Unfortunately so far there is no epidemiological evidence that CFS is due to an external poison. No plausibly damaging food item has been identified in the European diet. But it is impossible to disprove the possibility that some common article of food might have toxic effects in unlucky people with some particular genetic make-up.

Is the problem a low blood pressure and inadequately-filled blood circulation, due to lack of steroid hormones, possibly because of impaired function of the pituitary or adrenal glands? There has been intermittent interest in this possibility over several years, but it is disappointing that low dose cortisol (hydrocortisone) treatment produces improvement in symptoms which is only slight and hardly worthwhile because of the side-effects of suppressing patients' own adrenal gland function. Steroids have a definite non-specific tonic effect in some people. It remains unproven that CFS is due to pituitary or adrenal gland dysfunction.

Although CFS patients have normal electrocardiograms and normal heart function when they are resting, during exercise they have a reduced oxygen consumption and work capacity compared with matched healthy control subjects. Their maximum heart rate is greatly reduced. Muscle metabolism during exercise shows evidence of impaired energy supply. But an obvious problem in attributing reduced capacity for physical work to a muscle disorder is that it may simply result from prolonged inactivity as well as from reduced central nervous system drive. There is usually no good evidence of any specific muscle defect in CFS. In any case, it is difficult to see why a primary muscle disease should produce mental as well as physical fatigue.

Looking after patients with CFS is frustrating. A doctor can't explain to his patient the cause of the illness because he doesn't know what it is. He can't give any practical help. The condition often appears to be used as an excuse to give up work, either in the home or outside it, leaving spouse, partner, parent, friend or even child to cope as best they can. Some patients have already had an episode of major depression before the onset of CFS. Although the definition of CFS put forward by the Atlanta Center for Disease Control in the USA specifically excludes patients with major prior psychological illnesses, there are often minor psychological symptoms before CFS is diagnosed. Some doctors regard the illness as 'often a culturally sanctioned form of illness behavior'[4]. Faced with the evidence of a strong association between CFS and depression some physicians suggest that since depression is a psychological disorder, CFS is likely to be one also. But this argument overlooks strong evidence that severe depression, especially 'bipolar' depression (that kind which alternates with intervals of maniacal excitement) often responds much more successfully to manifestly 'organic' therapy such as lithium than to psychotherapy.

Central nervous system abnormalities

It is well-known that the rate of blood flow in different brain regions changes approximately in parallel with changes in the electrical and chemical metabolic activity of nerve cells in those regions. In CFS most outer (cortical) regions of the brain have reduced blood flow[5]. There is a general reduction in nerve activity, which is confirmed by other evidence of reduced local consumption of glucose and reduced uptake of oxygen. The rate of blood flow at the back of the brain (in the brain 'stem') is also reported to be reduced in CFS[6]. Apparent abnormalities have been reported in many series of patients having magnetic resonance imaging (MRI) of the brain. Although similar areas can be seen in normal people, they are much commoner in people with CFS[7], though not all investigators agree[8].

Some authors have attributed the symptoms of CFS to chronic habitual overbreathing, but this has been carefully checked and has not been confirmed as an important causal factor.

Is there a plausible unifying hypothesis?

No such hypothesis has yet achieved substantial acceptance. All have been lacking in detail. The first thing to say is that the condition has no obvious lethal consequences and there is no evidence to suggest that it might shorten life. (Most of my patients have been in their thirties or forties). So far I know of no post-mortem observations. There is often evidence that people with CFS have had previous depression and neurotic personality traits but too much can be made of this. It is only to be expected that a previous psychological disorder would aggravate any symptoms arising from a basic non-psychological cause. The presence of psychological disorder does not absolve us from looking further afield. We have to try to disentangle a possible underlying physical cause from its psychological overlay.

116

When I was first a medical student I was very keen on psychological explanations for physical symptoms. And I have sometimes had the gratifying experience of patients losing their physical symptoms after psychological counselling. For example, a male patient of mine came to recognise that hopeless marital incompatibility was his underlying problem, not a physical disease. His physical symptoms were immediately cured by divorce. A woman realised that her rejection of sex in her marriage, with consequent physical symptoms, derived from previous childhood sexual abuse by her father. I also recall a young recently-married woman running a low-grade fever, confirmed by two weeks' observation in hospital. Nothing was found after extensive tests. But the fever resolved after a simple operation to incise an imperforate hymen which had made intercourse impossible. So actual physical symptoms (genuine fever in this last case) can undoubtedly be caused by mental anxiety.

On the other hand I have just as often found physical explanations for apparently neurotic symptoms. When I was a junior doctor working long hours I began to have episodes of cramping central abdominal pain which I thought were probably due to stress and anxiety. They were immediately cured after I passed a round worm (*Ascaris lumbricoides*) in my stool and gave myself appropriate eradicatory treatment. This reminds me of a maxim that I have found surprisingly useful: a patient willing to accept a psychological explanation for bodily symptoms is probably suffering from a physical disorder; conversely, one who rejects the possibility of a psychological cause probably has one. This may sound nonsensical but any experienced physician can think of examples.

I recall vividly a 35-year-old woman who complained of sweating and indescribable sinking feelings after intercourse. The cause seemed to be the sexual habits of her husband who had to be first tied up, beaten and humiliated. This disgusted her. She had consulted psychiatrists without obtaining any satisfaction. A surgeon had removed some of her thyroid gland by an operation on her neck because her 'basal metabolic rate' was elevated, suggesting overactivity of the gland. Her blood pressure was normal and there was no apparent physical abnormality. I was in despair when, after leaving the ward, she returned to my outpatient clinic complaining of the same old symptoms. Unable to think of anything else useful to do, I sent a random urine specimen off to have adrenal gland hormones measured. She proved to have a vast excess of circulating adrenaline. After my surgical colleague Leslie LeQuesne had removed an adrenaline-secreting tumour the size of an orange from one of her adrenal glands she lost all her psychological as well as her physical symptoms.

Possible involvement of the reticular activating system

After reviewing as dispassionately as possible all the available evidence, I believe that a powerful case can be made that small localised defects in part of the upper brain stem, brought about in most cases by a previous virus infection, interfere with the ascending 'reticular activating system' (RAS) located at both sides of the brain stem (see Fig. 20). In animal experiments this has been shown to raise the level of electrical activity of the brain cortex when it is stimulated. Damage to the RAS diminishes arousal[9]. Brain imaging by positron emission tomography (PET) and by single photon emission computerised tomography (SPECT) shows that patients with depression as well as with CFS have reduced metabolic rate and local blood flow in many areas of the brain cortex, compared with normal subjects. But recent data suggest that it is only in CFS that brain stem metabolism is reduced, compared either with normal people or people with depression[10]. These observations fit well with previous work, already mentioned, of reduced brain stem blood flow in CFS[6]. They also fit with the hypothesis that the underlying functional defect in CFS is in

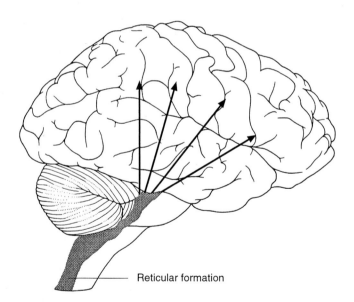

Figure 20 Diagram to show the general course of nerves comprising the reticular activating system, arising at the sides of the brain stem (extending over a considerable part of its length) and spreading forwards and upwards to make contact with the cerebral cortex.

the reticular formation of the brain stem. If all these observations are confirmed they might lead to the Holy Grail: an objective diagnostic test for CFS.

The syndrome of 'post-polio fatigue' is highly relevant. Fatigue disproportionate to neuromuscular paralysis was observed long ago after people had recovered from acute poliomyelitis[11]. It was present every day in these patients and increased as the day went on. Post-mortem data show damage in the region of the RAS and its cortical connections. The similarity of symptoms between post-polio fatigue and CFS is remarkable. Persistent damage to nerve cells, rather than simply the persistence of viruses at some site, seems a plausible explanation of fatigue and neurological dysfunction, as I have envisaged in a recent review[12].

A striking clinical feature of multiple sclerosis – a much-studied disease (see Chapter 3) – is fatigue, which is present in almost all cases. It often precedes any identifiable paralysis. My wife had noticed otherwise inexplicable fatigue, especially in hot weather, several years before she had any neurological symptoms or signs of MS. Later she developed a stiff (spastic) paralysis of the legs. The diagnosis of MS was confirmed by magnetic resonance imaging (MRI) of her brain. I have seen several patients whose initial symptoms of MS were ascribed to hysteria because nothing could initially be found on examination or after tests. No-one seriously suggests that fatigue in MS is psychological simply because it cannot yet be clearly attributed to lesions consistently found in any well-defined site in the brain. But multiple small lesions around the brain ventricles can almost invariably be demonstrated by MRI in MS (see Fig. 5, p. 23). It seems reasonable to suggest that they are in some way the cause of the characteristic fatigue.

At present it appears to be a tenable hypothesis to suggest:
1 that the defect consists of small, multiple, patchily distributed lesions affecting the ascending reticular activating system;
2 that the lesions may result from previous damage by an infective agent, probably an enterovirus, Epstein-Barr virus or herpesvirus-6, perhaps a rickettsial organism;
3 that the syndrome does not require living viruses necessarily to be present in the putative structural lesions, nor even for any active inflammation to be present;
4 that lack of activation of the cortex produces the sensation of fatigue without gross neurological abnormality, other than some defects in postural blood vessel control and giddiness.

Even if such a hypothesis proves that an initiating acute illness can only trigger CFS in people previously predisposed by their psychological make-up, there are enough clues to justify further studies. The identification of tangible lesions underlying CFS would be immensely valuable to patients, even if it led to no immediate therapeutic advance. And in the confusing scenario which CFS presents the identification of an organic basis for the illness would provide a more rational basis for therapy than exists at present.

I am hopeful that improved regional brain imaging and regional studies of brain metabolism may eventually answer the big question whether tangible brain stem lesions consistently underlie CFS. In that case its psychological manifestations could be the result of those lesions.

Alternatively, perhaps CFS is 'all in the mind', as many physicians believe. It makes a lot of difference who is right. My personal approach has been to say to patients: 'I don't know the cause of your chronic fatigue and I have found no evidence of serious disease in my examination or tests. In my experience most people with your condition gradually improve with time. ... Come and see me again in three months' time so that I can see how things are going. In the meantime, take as much exercise as you can as long as it is not making you too exhausted'. Rather more specific advice has been given by some psychiatrists who advocate 'cognitive behaviour therapy' which has had some success in a controlled clinical trial. But such successes do nothing to solve the problem of causation. We all know that extreme fatigue can be overcome by extreme effort of will. How can an observer ever know how much fatigue someone with CFS is experiencing and how hard they are trying to overcome it?

Summary

The chronic fatigue syndrome (CFS), sometimes incorrectly called 'myalgic encephalomyelitis' (ME), has been intensively studied during the last 40 years, but no conclusions have yet been agreed about its cause. Most cases nowadays are sporadic. In the established chronic condition there are no consistently abnormal physical signs or abnormalities on laboratory investigation. Many physicians remain convinced that the symptoms are psychological rather than physical in origin. This view is reinforced by the emotional way in which many patients present themselves. Furthermore, there is an overlap of symptoms between CFS and depression. This remains a source of confusion.

There is some evidence both for an active virus infection and for an immunological disorder in CFS. Many observations suggest that the syndrome might derive from residual damage to the reticular activating system (RAS) of the upper brain stem and to its cortical projections. Such damage could be produced by a previous infection, which is most likely to have been with a virus.

Studies by modern imaging techniques have not been entirely consistent, but many magnetic resonance imaging studies already suggest that small discrete patchy lesions can be found in the brain stem and in layers of cells just beneath the brain cortex. There is reduced blood flow in many regions of the brain, especially in the brain stem. Similar lesions have been reported after poliomyelitis and in multiple sclerosis, in both of which conditions chronic fatigue is characteristically present. In the well-known post-polio fatigue syndrome, lesions are mainly in the RAS of the brain stem and in its subcortical connections. If eventually similar underlying lesions in the RAS can be identified in CFS the therapeutic target for CFS would be better defined than it is at present. A number of logical approaches to treatment can already be envisaged.

13

INFLAMMATORY BOWEL DISEASE: ULCERATIVE COLITIS AND CROHN'S DISEASE

I am discussing these two conditions together, because it can be difficult and sometimes impossible to distinguish between them. 'Ulcerative colitis' (UC) is almost exclusively a disease of the lower part of the bowel (the colon and rectum) – the so-called 'large bowel'. The colon is a wide tube running in a loop from the lower right abdomen up, across and down to the lower left abdomen. It terminates in the wider rectum (Fig. 10, p. 51). Ulcerative 'col(on)itis' means that there is inflammation of the colon causing ulceration, though the disease invariably begins in the rectum. Food residues are mainly liquid when they enter the colon. The colon absorbs water and dries up the food residues, which are eventually passed into the rectum and out through the anus.

Crohn's disease (CD), named after the man who first recognised and described it, used to be called 'regional ileitis' because commonly the lower (more distal) part of the small bowel – the ileum – (see Fig. 10, p. 51) is inflamed. 'Crohn's disease' is now the preferred name because the disease can affect parts of the gut other than the ileum (see Fig. 21) and because its cause is still unknown. It has many features in common with UC. In both there is inflammation of the wall of the bowel, but inflammation in UC only affects the rectum and colon and is largely confined to the superficial (mucosal) layer of the bowel wall. In CD inflammatory changes extend throughout the entire thickness of the bowel wall. UC can be cured by surgical removal of the colon, but cutting out bits of gut affected by CD, though it may relieve symptoms for a year or two, seldom leads to permanent cure. The disease recurs in new sites and almost invariably at the junction of the two gut ends (the 'anastomosis'). With each operation to remove some of the small intestine, its absorptive capacity is reduced. Widespread CD can threaten life simply through failure to absorb enough food. In days before permanent artificial feeding had become a practical proposition I once had the devastating experience of helplessly watching one of my patients, a young man with extensive CD and multiple surgical resections, slowly and inexorably starve to death.

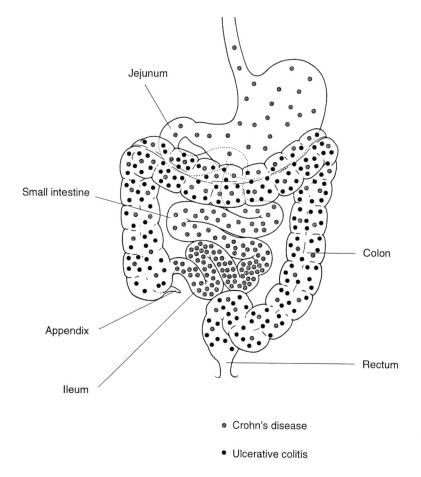

Jejunum

Small intestine

Colon

Appendix

Rectum

Ileum

⊘ Crohn's disease

● Ulcerative colitis

Figure 21 Diagram of the gut showing parts involved by Crohn's disease and by ulcerative colitis. Crohn's disease can affect any part of the gut, though predominantly the ileum; ulcerative colitis exclusively affects the large bowel.

In both conditions there are all the changes of inflammation (see p. 11). The bowel lining may become ulcerated, leading to bleeding. Pain may occur anywhere in either condition, but is commonly felt in the central lower abdomen in UC. In CD it is often felt in the right lower abdomen where it may mimic grumbling appendicitis. In UC there is often bright red blood in the stool. In CD the bleeding tends to be of lesser degree, but may lead to iron deficiency anaemia. In addition, the involvement of the last part of the small intestine in CD can interfere with the absorption of vitamin B_{12}. This can lead to a different type of anaemia.

124

Under the microscope all the changes of inflammation may be seen in both conditions, though in CD there may also be tiny pale granules (granulomata) in the bowel wall. These resemble the 'tubercles' characteristic of tuberculosis. The history of smoking is interesting. Cigarette smoking is a definite precipitating factor for CD, whereas smoking seems to be protective against UC, possibly because one of the constituents of tobacco smoke increases the production of protective mucus by the lining of the colon. Nicotine has even been used therapeutically in ulcerative colitis. Despite these differences, it is often difficult to distinguish the two conditions because parts of the colon may be affected by CD lesions, with typical granulomata. This can give rise to symptoms identical with those of UC, a situation described as 'Crohn's colitis'. When only the colon is affected by inflammatory changes, classification is impossible in about 15% of cases. However, when disease does not initially appear in the rectum, the condition can be confidently identified as Crohn's colitis.

Steroids are the most effective drugs for inducing remission in either condition, but their use is limited by side-effects which include muscle and bone weakness, high blood pressure, diabetes and trunk obesity. In UC, steroid therapy can be given by enemas. This reduces absorption into the body, with consequently fewer side-effects than with oral administration. It is doubtful whether the newer steroids (e.g. budesonide) are superior to standard steroids such as prednisone. They are certainly much more expensive.

The early symptoms of UC are similar to those of irritable bowel syndrome (IBS) discussed in Chapter 6. There is often lower abdominal pain with frequent loose stools or diarrhoea. But in IBS, by definition, there is no inflammation present in the wall of the bowel and there is no ulceration. In both UC and CD there is loss of the normal thin lining layer of cells, the bowel 'epithelium'. (Incidentally, this word has an interesting Greek derivation, from 'epi-' = above/upon and 'thele' = nipple. It was chosen to emphasise the thinness of the lining layer of cells, resembling the thin skin overlying the nipple.)

Epidemiology

The prevalence of UC in Europe and the USA is about 150 per 100,000 population, so UC is a not uncommon disease. The number of newly-diagnosed cases is about 10 per 100,000 population annually. CD is slightly less common and its prevalence is about 100 in every 100,000. White races are more commonly affected by CD than black. Young adults (15–40) are the most common victims of both diseases, which are typically diagnosed some ten months after the first symptoms appear.

Genetics

There is at least a 10% risk of developing UC for anyone with a first degree relative with UC or CD. The risk is higher for CD than UC. If someone has an identical twin with CD he or she will have around a 40% chance of also getting the disease, whereas the chances for non-identical twins are only a few percent. Most surveys suggest that several genes determine susceptibility to both CD and UC and that some are common to both conditions. There seem to be genes on chromosomes 16 and 12 which may determine whether someone will develop inflammatory bowel disease (IBD) or not. But environmental trigger factors are at least as important, probably more so.

Cause

Identifying the cause of human diseases often advances quickly when there is an example of the same condition in animals. Unfortunately spontaneous IBD in animals is very rare. The ideal animal model has not yet been found, though the surgically-created 'ileal pouch disease' has many features in common with IBD and certainly suggests that bacteria play a big part in the inflammatory process. Long-standing inflammatory changes in the gut wall of animals can be induced by a variety of external damaging agents. The general topic of IBD has been the subject of several useful reviews[1].

The way that UC starts in the rectum makes one think that perhaps an infecting organism gains access to the large bowel from the anal orifice, from which it spreads upwards. In early cases there may be a clear line of demarcation between the lower inflamed bowel wall and the upper unaffected part. (This finding normally suggests that a trial of local medical rather than surgical treatment should be the first step.) It remains a complete mystery why whatever causes UC never ascends to the gut above the colon. Is this because of the inborn structural difference between colon and lower small intestine (ileum)? Or is the difference chemical or bacteriological?

Many chronic (i.e. long-standing) diseases such as multiple sclerosis and rheumatoid arthritis (see Chapters 3 and 8) have a strong association with certain human leucocyte antigen (HLA: see p. 27) groups. A strong HLA association suggests that the condition may be one of the so-called 'infective/immune' group of diseases in which an external infecting agent so closely resembles some human tissue or organ that the circulating antibodies and defensive lymphocytes which the body produces to combat the infection react in a damaging way against body tissues or organs. HLA associations have been sought in IBD, but have not yet convincingly been found.

Does infection initiate IBD?

I have already mentioned in Chapter 6 the complex microbial environment of the gut, especially the large bowel. The sudden way in which IBD often begins suggests that it may be initiated by an intercurrent infection, or by some damaging dietary or microbial product. But neither in CD nor UC is there consistent evidence of any infecting organism. The affected gut wall becomes more permeable to bacterial toxins and even to living bacteria (so-called 'translocation'), but whether this is cause or effect is unclear. Sulfasalazine has antibiotic activity and is useful in treatment, but probably works more as a suppressor of the inflammatory reaction rather than something which kills an infecting organism. Its active principle (5-aminosalicylic acid) is an aspirin-like drug. Attempts have been made to implicate the measles virus in CD, raising the possibility that measles vaccination, especially the use of the 'measles, mumps and rubella' (MMR) vaccine might predispose to Crohn's disease as well as to other conditions later in life. This has been a most unfortunate scare story. The suggestion arose because an apparent excess of inflammatory bowel disease was observed in people previously vaccinated against measles, compared with unvaccinated ones. There are so many possibilities of the two groups being dissimilar (e.g. in respect of diet, social class, geographical district and attending doctors) that the results come under the strong suspicion of the statistical fault known as 'confounding'. The direct evidence for the relationship is poor. Tests for measles virus in CD tissues have drawn a blank.

The suddenness of onset in many cases of IBD might be explained by the affected individual meeting for the first time a particular 'antigen' (see p. 27). If this was not a constituent of an infecting organism, it might perhaps have been an article of diet, acting as a trigger to set off a chain of immune reactions which then become self-sustaining. We do not know what the antigen might be, though many possible candidates have been suggested. Cyclosporine, an immunosuppressive drug, improves symptoms in CD by inhibiting the production by specialised 'T-lymphocytes' (see p. 26) of damaging cytokines such as IL-2 and IL-6. Its effectiveness strongly suggests that there has been a harmful activation of the immune system.

Considerable improvement has been obtained in CD (e.g. in closing gut-to-skin fistulas) by giving antibodies which neutralise damaging cytokines such as 'TNFα', which is present in large amounts in and around inflammatory cells in the gut wall. Trials are now in progress to evaluate antibodies to yet another cytokine, IL-12. The improvement brought about by giving antibodies to TNFα has been compared with that obtainable by the same treatment in rheumatoid arthritis (RA) (see p. 74). But as in that condition, antibodies tend to develop to the antibody. Its benefits are therefore limited. By analogy with RA anti-TNFα probably needs to be given together with low-dose methotrexate(see p. 74). Interleukin-1(IL-1) is another cytokine which has also been strongly associated with damaging inflammatory reactions in IBD.

Clearly many different inflammation-producing cytokines are involved in CD. By analogy with asthma (see Chapter 2), the transcription factor NFκB is a potentially attractive target for inhibitory therapy because it controls synthesis of so many cytokines. Several trials are under way.

There is much genetic diversity in the way in which different people react to damaging cytokines. This may account for differing individual susceptibilities to CD or UC. Despite considerable success in controlling symptoms, no anti-cytokine therapy has so far produced improvement which continues after treatment has stopped. Several groups of investigators have tried to identify some genetic factor which predisposes to IBD (e.g. defects in a DNA repair gene). Minor degrees of predisposition have been noted for certain articles of diet and for some common intercurrent infections. The associations are too weak to suggest that they are important causes of either CD or UC, though the consumption of margarine has been rather strongly associated with UC in a recent Japanese study[2]. The problem about this sort of study is statistical. If the consumption of a large number of individual items of food is related to their apparent associations with IBD it is inevitable that some relationships will be discovered which seem to be more than chance occurrences. At best such studies can only be used as pilots for larger surveys which concentrate on the association of interest.

CD is often associated with what seem to be immunological complications in organs outside the gut (e.g. inflammation of joints, skin and eyeballs). These observations raise the possibility that the disease is triggered by infection with a ubiquitous bacterium, to which only certain unfortunate individuals are susceptible. There is certainly a genetic element in susceptibility to CD and it might be of this nature. Susceptibility might lie in defective function of the lining cell layers of the gut, or in the nature of the immunological response to damaging material entering the gut wall.

Because the granulomata seen in the intestinal wall in CD resemble those seen in tuberculosis, searches have often been made in microscope sections of bowel wall for tubercle bacilli, but none has been seen or grown in culture. There are close resemblances between segments of DNA detected in CD tissue and DNA extracted from a paratuberculosis bacterium related to the tubercle bacillus itself. One such organism is the paratuberculosis mycobacterium which causes Johne's disease, an inflammatory granulomatous condition of the gut in ruminants. This is an exciting observation; but unfortunately the same DNA code has been found in normal people and in other conditions. Other similar investigations have proved entirely negative. This is an area which cries out for resolution between opposing research camps. Perhaps the organism needs to infect a susceptible person to cause disease and is perhaps harmless to most people. This is no means an uncommon situation. For example, most of the adult population of the UK have been exposed to, and infected by, the Epstein-Barr virus in childhood, without suffering any serious disease. But when susceptible young adults get infected they can develop the disease recognised as glandular fever, as I mentioned in Chapter 8.

Although currently used anti-tuberculosis drugs are ineffective in CD, some success has recently been achieved with drugs which have been shown to be effective against the paratuberculosis bacterium. If I had to bet at present I would put my money on the cause of CD, and possibly of UC as well, being an acquired infection by a paratuberculosis organism.

Could the blood supply of the gut be important?

I have a particular personal reason for wondering whether the blood supply of the gut might be of some importance, perhaps by making the gut more vulnerable to infection. Some 25 years ago I made the diagnosis of CD in a young woman. Some years later I was consulted by her sister, who was complaining of rather vague abdominal pain associated with eating. When I examined her abdomen I heard a regular rushing noise over the upper abdomen in time with each beat of the heart. Our professor of surgery was also impressed by this. He arranged an angiogram (an X-ray taken after arterial injection of contrast material) of the superior mesenteric artery. This showed very severe narrowing of the main artery supplying all the small intestine and quite a lot of the large intestine. Blood tests had provided no evidence of inflammation such as is usually seen in CD. The erthrocyte sedimentation rate (ESR) – a test for inflammation – was normal. But while further tests were awaited the woman developed what appeared to be acute appendicitis. The excised appendix showed under the microscope typical changes of CD. My surgical colleague and I had official complaints lodged against both of us by the family for failing to diagnose the condition earlier.

At that time I had no knowledge that CD could be associated with premature atheromatous disease making the large arteries narrow; but there has since been some evidence of the association. This experience made me wonder at the time, and since, whether possibly a poor blood supply can make the bowel wall less resistant to bacterial or virus invasion. This could be relevant if CD is started by an infection. Second infections with *Mycobacterium tuberculosis* (the bacterium which causes human tuberculosis) are usually found in the apices of the lungs – the upper parts, where blood supply is poor. In days before streptomycin and other specific antibiotics became available, bed rest was the cornerstone of antituberculous treatment. It is now thought to work by increasing the amount of blood going to the upper parts of the lungs.

Another reason for speculating that the gut's blood supply may be important is the almost invariable recurrence of CD at the site of the join (anastomosis) when a segment of small intestine has been cut out. It seems likely that at this region the blood supply could have been damaged by the previous surgery.

Responses to therapy in IBD

There are differences in the response to therapy in CD and UC. Dietary control and certain antibiotics (notably metronidazole) are helpful in CD but not in UC. Aminosalicylates such as sulphsalazine are useful in UC but rather less so in CD. Apart from steroids, which help anyway by increasing mucus synthesis, other immunosuppressants such as azathioprine, methotrexate, cyclosporine and mycophenolate may be useful but carry risks of their own. The merits and dangers of each new immunosuppressant drug has to be assessed in careful clinical trials against the 'gold standards' provided by azathioprine and methotrexate. As in many other fields, the rate of discovery of new drugs vastly exceeds the rate at which each can be critically evaluated against the others.

Psychological factors (e.g. anxiety and depression) are sometimes invoked as potential causes of IBD. Psychotherapy has been tried, particularly in UC, though with little success. Anyone who has seen, as I have, many patients with UC before and after surgical removal of

130

the diseased bowel will find it difficult to believe that psychological disturbance is an important cause of the condition. Patients are anxious, but this is only to be expected for such a disabling and unpleasant condition.

Summary

Ulcerative colitis (UC) and Crohn's disease (CD) are both relatively common inflammatory conditions of the gut. UC affects the colon, but CD mainly the lower small intestine, but also other parts of the gut. Both conditions cause substantial constitutional symptoms as well as diarrhoea and abdominal pain. UC can be permanently cured by removal of the colon. Removal of the whole small intestine for CD is not feasible because of its essential absorptive function. Both conditions can be improved, though not cured, by immunosuppressive therapy.

It is difficult to summarise a host of different views about the cause of CD and UC, but a reasonable synthesis might be along the following lines: first the gut wall is attacked either by an infecting organism or an external toxin; this leads to increased permeability of the gut wall to many other damaging materials; if the patient has the appropriate genetic susceptibility to cytokines (inflammation mediators) the inflammation becomes self-perpetuating. Immune reactions may then affect other tissues outside the gut, especially in CD.

CD and UC are distinct diseases, almost certainly having different triggers, but sharing many attributes in common, especially reactions to damaging cytokines.

14

MIGRAINE

The word 'migraine' seems to have been derived from a corruption of '(he)micrainia' (something affecting one half of the cranium). It is a very common condition, affecting 20% of women and 15% of men at some time in their lives. It is commonest in early adult life, though first attacks often occur before the age of 10. It may be diagnosed retrospectively by talking to intelligent and observant older children. As sufferers grow up attacks become less frequent. Migraine is rare in the elderly. A recent review is a useful summary[1].

Its manifestations are varied. Typically it is a specific type of episodic headache with a small set of associated neurological symptoms. Classic attacks, experienced by a quarter of migraine sufferers, begin with an 'aura' (Latin: breeze, smell or gleam of light). This usually takes the form of a so-called 'fortification spectrum', in which there appears to be a curved horizontal ridge of a zig-zag pattern in front of the eyes. The sufferer usually describes it as looking through a heat haze. The aura lasts for 20–40 minutes and may be followed by a headache lasting 12–48 hours if it is not treated. The headache is often initially confined to one side of the head. It may be associated with nausea, sometimes vomiting, and very occasionally with abdominal pain. The aura with its fortification spectrum may occur without the succeeding headache. Or headaches may occur without any preceding aura, as happens in the majority of cases. A third of migraine sufferers have experienced both types of presentation. During the visual aura there may be short-lived neurological defects, such as temporary paralysis of skeletal muscles, or curious localised changes or defects in sensation. The extraordinary condition of transient global amnesia is thought usually to be a manifestation of migraine.

The neurological signs accompanying the headache are normally transient. Recovery is usually complete, though a severe attack of 'hemiplegic migraine' (migraine accompanied by paralysis down one side of the body) may leave a permanent disturbance of function. One of my patients, a man of 19, had a well-marked partial paralysis on one side of his body which persisted for many weeks after he had otherwise recovered from a particularly severe attack. It is not too surprising, therefore, that very occasionally migraine sufferers have experienced persisting disturbances of movement, balance, vision or hearing. These presumably reflect actual damage either to a brain pathway, or to the eye or inner ear during an attack.

Treatments for migraine

It is worth reviewing briefly the currently available treatments for the light this might throw on the nature of the disease. Migraine is initially managed with aspirin or paracetamol, perhaps with an anti-vomiting drug. More powerful and specific treatments fall into two main groups: relievers and preventers.

For relief, the first really effective drug has been sumatriptan, which is a serotonin agonist, i.e. a drug which mimics the effects of the natural hormone serotonin. It works best when given by injection under the skin, though is moderately effective by mouth. Many other similar compounds such as naratriptan and zolmitriptan have been introduced. 'Triptans' are thought to act on specialised serotonin receptors in brain artery walls, causing constriction of those arteries. These drugs work quickly and provide fast relief of headache for 80% of sufferers in 2–4 hours. Although serotonin itself is a small simple chemical molecule, it can react with many different receptors and perform many different functions. Seven major types and eight sub-types of serotonin receptor have already been identified within the central nervous system. It seems certain that many other drugs will be introduced in the future.

'Preventer' drugs include pizotifen (Sanomigran) and methysergide. 'Beta blockers' like propranolol are thought to work by stabilising cerebral blood vessels. They occasionally induce a permanent cure after several courses of treatment.

Cause

About 70% of migraine sufferers have a first degree relative (parent, sister or brother) who also has migraine. But migraine is so common anyway that many apparent examples of heredity may simply be due to chance. The disease does not occur in any simple 'Mendelian' proportions[*]. The shared environment of family members could be as

[*] The laws of heredity were discovered in the 19th century by Gregor Mendel, an

important as inheritance. This may be specially relevant in families whose migraine is not associated with an aura. Such cases may be sometimes best classified as 'recurrent tension headache' rather than true migraine. A large study of adult twin pairs in Finland compared the coincidence of migraine in identical and non-identical twins. This allowed the genetic contribution to migraine to be accurately estimated. It varied between 34% and 51% in different migraine types. There is some evidence to suggest that migraine accompanied by an aura is strongly genetically determined, with first degree relatives having a fourfold risk of the condition in comparison with people unrelated to a migraine sufferer. A specific chromosomal mutation has been identified in 25% of Japanese sufferers from this variety of migraine. Migraine attacks without an associated aura may be fundamentally different from classic migraine; it is notable that spouses of sufferers are often affected.

One identifiable biochemical difference between people with the two types of migraine has been reported. Superoxide dismutase (SOD) is a natural cellular enzyme. It is found in many places, but particularly in the blood platelets, where it may give protection against oxidative stress. In typical classic migraine with aura, the blood concentration of SOD is reduced[2].

> A marker for the rare condition of familial hemiplegic migraine (FHM) (an autosomal dominant condition) appears to be on chromosome 19p13. A minor faulty gene on the same chromosome could perhaps contribute to the inheritance of other types of migraine, though such a link has only rarely been reported. The mutation causing FHM seems to affect a gene coding for voltage-sensitive 'calcium channels' in brain cells[3]. These have been categorised as of the 'P/Q' type and are distinct from those involved in blood vessel function. The entry of calcium into cells through sub-microscopic calcium channels is a trigger which switches on many cell functions. FHM seems to be associated with a sudden reduction in blood flow starting at the back of the brain. Some defect in the control of the entry of calcium into the muscle cells lining the brain arteries might lead to the arterial constriction and the subsequent dilation which are probably the basis for a typical migraine attack.

Austrian monk of the Augustinian order who became Abbot of Brünn. Working methodically in the monastery garden with both edible and sweet peas, he recognised types of inheritance to which he gave the names 'dominant' and 'recessive'. He also recognised in cross-pollinated ('hybrid') peas that their offspring showed different characters in well-defined mathematical proportions. His observations passed unnoticed for many years, but he is now recognised as the father of genetics. He was an original scientist who ranks with the very greatest.

Prevalence of migraine is remarkably constant in developed countries. Approximately 6% of men and 15% of women are affected. Symptoms typically begin in the teens, and diminish in frequency and severity after middle age. In people with active migraine, attacks typically come every two to three weeks and last about a day. Migraine attacks are often related to the menstrual cycle in women and usually remit during pregnancy. Head trauma has often led to precipitation of attacks of migrainous headaches which can usually be treated effectively by anti-migraine drugs. Diet has often been invoked as a precipitating cause of migraine, usually through an allergic response to certain foods.

The two main current hypotheses of the causation of migraine are the vascular spasm model, and the spreading cortical depression hypothesis. Most researchers believe that the aura of migraine has a different cause from the headache. Certainly the two can be separated as I can testify from my own experience. I have had several episodes of typical visual aura with a fortification spectrum, each lasting about 30 minutes, but I have never had any succeeding headache.

Most people believe that migraine headache is due to dilation of some of the main brain arteries, which grossly look like Fig. 22. Regional blood flow is presumed to be diminished during the aura, though I have not been able to find direct observations of this. There is general agreement that cerebral blood flow is increased during the headache phase of an attack. This would fit with the striking relief of headache by sumatriptan, which is a drug which selectively constricts blood vessels in the head.

The vascular spasm model

A point in favour of vascular spasm causing reduced local cerebral blood flow perfusion is that there have been well-documented cases of intermittent monocular blindness leading, after many years of attacks, to permanent blindness of the affected eye, accompanied by reduced calibre of all the retinal arteries. 'Infarction' (death of tissue caused by inadequate blood supply) of the retina has been occasionally seen in migraine. This has apparently been caused by temporary closure of the central retinal artery. If an attack of migraine is precipitated by constriction of brain arteries it is natural to ask whether there is any evidence of circulating constrictor chemicals in the blood of migraine sufferers. Cytokines such as 'substance-P' and 'neurokinin-1' have

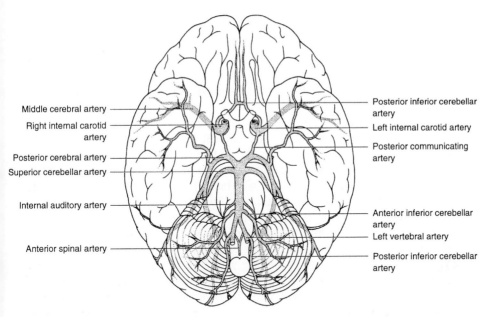

Figure 22 Main arteries at the base of the brain, viewed from below after removing the brain from the skull.

been looked for, but have yet to be assigned a definite causal role. Nor has serotonin, even though sumatriptan is an effective treatment for the migraine headache and can reduce cerebral blood flow in some conditions in which it is increased.

Constriction of blood vessels could also be due to reduction in the concentration of some dilating material. The best-known is a simple gas (nitric oxide) which contains one atom each of nitrogen and oxygen. However, nitric oxide is more likely to be relevant to migraine as a potential dilator chemical causing headache. Its antagonist 'L-NAME' has been reported to alleviate migrainous headache.

A minor point in favour of the vascular model is that freestyle ice skaters who spin a lot get more frequent migraine attacks than ice dancers, who don't spin[4].

The spreading cortical depression hypothesis

Fits or seizures (epileptic attacks) are due to uncontrolled electrical excitation spreading over the brain. Epilepsy often starts from a small previously damaged area of the brain surface. One subject of hot

137

debate is whether migraine might result from similarly spreading electrical excitation, soon succeeded by 'spreading cortical depression'. An association between epilepsy and migraine has been firmly established and is not due to shared genetic susceptibility. In between attacks, migraine sufferers have been reported to have increased electrical excitability of the brain surface, though there is no agreement about its cause.

Electrical excitability has been measured in an interesting way through the intact skull, by magnetic stimulation. Michael Faraday recognised that changing magnetic fields generate currents in electrical conductors. So if a powerful magnetic field around the head is suddenly switched on, or suddenly changes direction, small electric currents are generated in conducting tissues in the brain. When the nerve tissues thus stimulated control muscle movement an objective measurement can be made of the electrical excitability of the brain surface.

There is some evidence that the brain stem as well as the brain cortex may play a part in initiating migraine attacks. However, a clear causal link between neuronal excitation and brain stem blood flow changes has yet to be firmly established.

Other hypotheses

One is that vascular spasm and spreading cortical depression might be linked through a vicious circle perpetuated by a local rise in the concentration of potassium, the element specially concerned with nervous electrical activity. This could be initiated either by localised intense nervous activity or by a transient reduction in local blood flow to a small area of the brain cortex. A local rise in potassium concentration could cause spasm of small arteries, local reduction of blood flow and the start of a vicious circle.

Blood platelets have come under suspicion as playing some part in migraine. Platelets are concerned in blood clotting and temporary aggregation of platelets has been well established as a cause of the so-called 'transient ischaemic attack' (TIA) – a sort of temporary stroke. However, aspirin, which reduces platelet stickiness and gives some protection against coronary artery thrombosis and against TIAs has little protective effect against migraine, though it gives some relief of headache.

Another possibility is that migraine could result from an 'axon reflex' which sends nerve impulses in the wrong direction, causing inflammation of the dura (the tough membrane covering the brain). This possibility arises because nerves conveying sensation to the brain sometimes have many branches, so that a sensory signal coming from one area can get routed backwards in another nerve branch to inflame a different area. This bizarre situation is well recognised in the skin. Impulses running backwards in nerves ordinarily conveying sensation can cause inflammation and a red flare in undamaged areas of skin surrounding a damaged area. Migraine has often been noted to be associated with sinusitis and with dental disease, either of which could be sending signals up branching sensory nerves to the brain, creating the possibility of a damaging axon reflex.

The 'trigger' which switches on a migraine attack has been looked for but has not so far been convincingly identified. There is suggestive evidence that gut infection with the bacterium *Helicobacter pylori*, an organism associated with peptic ulcer, may be a trigger. Some protection against recurrent migraine attacks has been reported to follow eradication of this bacterium from the gut.

It is remotely possible that the basic defect initiating an attack of migraine is local dilation of brain arteries. This definitely occurs during the headache phase. But if so why should this sometimes lead to permanent damage which appears to be due to a local reduction of blood flow? Could excessive arterial dilation at one site lead to a reduction in local blood pressure and hence flow at another site? We need good surveys of local brain blood flow distribution during the migraine aura, to see whether there is simply a reduction in overall cerebral blood flow, or whether there is evidence of unequal excess perfusion in one area causing underperfusion in other areas. It would be interesting to know what the total cerebral blood flow is during the early phase of a migraine attack, but I have not been able to find information about this.

Summary

Migraine is an extremely common condition which usually appears in early adult life and gets less common later. Classic migraine has two well-defined phases. One is associated with loss of function, most probably due to spasm of arteries supplying affected parts of the brain. This is associated with a sensory aura, usually visual. The later phase comprises a headache, typically covering one side of the head only. This phase is almost certainly associated with, and probably caused by, excessive dilation of arteries. The best treatment remedies are those which mimic the constrictor effect of serotonin, a drug which acts on brain arteries. It is not known at present whether recurrent, otherwise inexplicable, headaches not accompanied by an aura, are the same disease as classic migraine.

Although the migraine aura has for years been thought to be due to spasm of brain arteries, and the succeeding headache from dilation of the same arteries, attention is now being increasingly focused on electrical activity of nerve cells. There is a relation between migraine and epilepsy. This may be related to changed electrical excitability of nerve cells in the brain, associated with changes in cell membrane properties in respect of ions of certain chemical elements, especially calcium and potassium. We do not know whether an attack of migraine starts with a spreading electrical excitation followed by depression over the brain surface. This could produce first a consequent increase in local blood flow which would be followed by a decrease. Alternatively, the whole sequence of events might be triggered by initial spasm of certain brain arteries. Fortunately many of these questions will soon be answered as the techniques for non-invasive investigation of brain function improve.

15

HIGH BLOOD PRESSURE: 'ESSENTIAL' HYPERTENSION

I have found this chapter the most difficult to write. My main life's work in medical research has been trying to find the cause of so-called 'essential' hypertension. During my search I have come to hold strong opinions which most fellow scientists in the field do not share. I have probably failed to be fair to rival views. So readers of this chapter need to keep an open mind and realise that a bigot is trying to persuade them of his own interpretations. But let me start with a few facts.

Anatomy of the circulation

The simplest way to think about the circulation is that blood goes round the body in a figure-of-eight racetrack. The smaller loop is the lung ('pulmonary') circulation, the larger comprises the rest of the body (the 'systemic' circulation). Although the heart lies at the crossing of the two blood circuits, and the two sides of the heart contract and pump at the same time, there is normally no connection between them in the heart itself (Fig. 23).

To describe a circuit one can start anywhere. Let's start with the aorta, the main and largest artery in the body. In the adult it is an inch or more in diameter (3cm) where it leaves the heart. Blood flows to all the body tissues (e.g. brain, gut and muscles) through a set of large arteries. These branch repeatedly in all the organs they supply, finishing in a network of very small blood vessels (capillaries) which take nutrients to the tissues and remove waste products from them. Capillaries are tubes only about 1/2000 of an inch (8–20 microns) in diameter. They are too small to see with the naked eye and their internal diameter is only slightly larger than the red cells of the blood.

Blood is collected from the tissues by veins. The two largest veins (the venae cavae) convey blood into the right side of the heart. The larger veins contain flap valves which allow blood to flow only one

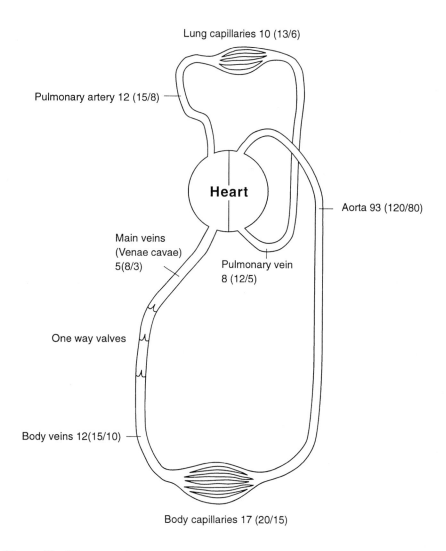

Lung capillaries 10 (13/6)

Pulmonary artery 12 (15/8)

Heart

Aorta 93 (120/80)

Main veins
(Venae cavae)
5(8/3)

Pulmonary vein
8 (12/5)

One way valves

Body veins 12(15/10)

Body capillaries 17 (20/15)

Figure 23 Diagram of the two main parts of the circulation, with the typical pressures at each point in a supine subject, in mmHg. The mean pressure is followed by typical values for pressure oscillations, in brackets, also in mmHg.

way, towards the heart. It was by study of these valves in human arm veins some 350 years ago that William Harvey realised that blood had to go round in a circuit. It did not simply oscillate with each heart beat, as people had previously believed.

From the right side of the heart blood is pumped through the pulmonary artery into the two lungs. The air we breathe in and out comes into contact with a fine network of very small blood vessels, the pulmonary capillaries. These surround the tiny air sacs (the alveoli: (see p. 5)). After going through the lungs blood is collected into the left 'atrium' (Latin: entrance hall) of the heart. Then it enters the main pumping chamber of the heart, the left 'ventricle' (Latin: 'ventriculus' = little stomach), and starts its journey round again. At its fastest it takes about 20 seconds for a complete circuit, and maybe only half that during strenuous exercise. But it could take a minute or two for a single blood cell to go round the circuit if it happened to be going a long distance and through a tissue with only a small blood supply (e.g. the bones of the foot).

An adult body contains about 9 pints (5 litres) of blood. More than 90% of this is in the systemic circulation, mainly in the veins and arteries, though a small amount is in the capillaries. The left side of the heart (the left atrium and left ventricle) does most of the work because it pumps blood up to a high pressure. The right side only has to pump blood through the lungs, which normally present very little resistance to flow: but see Chapter 18.

Pressures of blood in different parts of the circuit

All parts of the systemic circulation contain blood at a higher pressure than that in the corresponding parts of the pulmonary circulation. Stephen Hales (an English clergyman) directly measured systemic arterial blood pressure in a horse in 1733. He restrained the animal and tied a long tube into an artery. Blood rushed up the tube to reach a height of about six feet.

Physicists measure pressure in international standard (SI: système internationale) units such as kiloPascals (kPa). But for more than a century doctors have measured pressure in arteries by comparing it with the pressure generated by a vertical column of mercury. This metal, 13 times heavier than blood, is fluid at room temperature and more convenient than using a column of blood. Indeed, Stephen Hales himself made use of a mercury manometer to measure fluid pressures in plants. The 'sphygmomanometer' is used to measure indirectly the pressure in the main arm artery. (The name is derived from Greek: 'sphygmos' = pulse; 'manos' = rare, thin; 'metron' = measure.) A high air pressure is applied to a cuff around the upper arm, then the pressure is gently lowered until the pulse returns to the wrist or until a pulsating rushing noise can be heard by a stethoscope pressed against the main artery below the cuff. At this point the peak or 'systolic' (Greek: 'systolo' = contraction) pressure can be read off a graduated column of mercury or from some other pressure-measuring device, since it will be the same as the air pressure in the cuff.

Ironically, doctors and hospitals are now abandoning the mercury pressure measurer because mercury gives off a poisonous vapour even at room temperature. In a glass manometer this is harmless, but mercury manometers get abandoned and broken. The mercury trickles into flooring and crevices so that the level of mercury vapour in the air of hospitals and laboratories can become a real health hazard. The European Union is in process of banning this use of mercury. But so well established is the 'millimetres of mercury' unit for blood pressure measurement and so many mercury manometers remain in use all over the world that it will be decades before standard SI units of pressure (kPa) take over. It will be longer still before all mercury manometers are phased out. But so long as people remain familiar with the unique physical properties of mercury they will probably continue to find it easier to relate arterial blood pressure to the pressure exerted by a mercury column rather than train themselves to think and talk about kiloPascals.

In a normal adult the systolic pressure is about 120 millimetres of mercury, abbreviated to 'mmHg' because 'Hg' is the chemical symbol for mercury (itself an abbreviation of the expressive Latin: 'hydrargyrus' = water-silver). This pressure corresponds to about 16.5 kPa above the atmospheric pressure. That is only about one tenth the pressure in an average mains water tap. When the heart's left ventricle relaxes after discharging its contents into the arteries the pressure falls to a trough level, called the 'diastolic' (Greek: 'diastole' = dilation) pressure. This is around 80mmHg, or 11kPa. It is detected because of the disappearance of the pulse sound heard via the stethoscope over an arm artery as the cuff pressure in the upper arm is gradually lowered. Doctors conventionally write down the two pressures in shorthand as, for example, '120/80'. Because of the triangular shape of the pressure curve, the diastolic pressure is closer than the systolic pressure to the true average arterial pressure. The best estimate of mean pressure is given by adding one third of the pulse pressure (the difference between systolic and diastolic pressures) to the diastolic pressure. For a blood pressure of 120/80 the mean pressure is:

$$80 + \frac{120-80}{3} = 93 \text{ mmHg}$$

In the fine capillaries of the body the pressure is much lower, 15–20 mmHg on average. In the veins the pressure is lower still. It is often possible to see pulsation in the large veins of the neck of someone lying flat because the pressure there oscillates just above and below atmospheric pressure. It is amusing to look closely at the side of the neck in films or television dramas which show a supposed 'corpse' at close quarters. In some of them venous pulsation gives the game away.

The right atrium collects the blood from the great veins and pumps it into the right ventricle, which raises the average pressure to around 10–15 mmHg. This is normally high enough to send blood through the low resistance path of the lungs.

Systemic hypertension

'Hypertension' is a hybrid word (Greek: 'hyper-' = over, above; Latin: 'tens-' = stretch). Unless otherwise specified, the term always refers to the systemic circulation and to pressure in the large systemic arteries. Many surveys of whole populations have shown a frequency distribution of blood pressures, at rest, which look like Fig. 24. With increasing age of a population the average pressure increases, and there is a wider spread of pressures between individuals. In addition the frequency distribution curves become progressively skewed towards the right in the older age groups. Fig. 24 shows that there is no clear dividing line between high and low pressures. People with pressures consistently maintained above about 140/90 are described as 'hypertensive'. If this definition is used, about 4% of young adults in most developed countries are hypertensive. The proportion rises with age. By the age of 60 the definition includes about half the population, and by the age of 75 about 65%. The great majority of people in their seventies have a systolic pressure considerably greater than 140 mmHg. Despite the apparent normality of raised blood pressure in the older members of the community, hypertension is not a harmless variation at any age. On average, people's lifespan is inversely proportional to their blood pressure. People with blood pressures of 160/100 are much more likely than those with pressures of 120/80 mmHg to get arterial complications such as heart or kidney disease and strokes in later life. They will die younger. At the extreme end, a man whose blood pressure is at, say, 300/180 (which is about the highest pressure ever seen) is likely to die soon, within a month or two, probably from a brain haemorrhage, unless he is treated by blood-pressure-lowering drugs.

I am only talking about maintained hypertension. When a normal person engages in strenuous exercise, especially so-called isometric exercise like lifting heavy weights, the blood pressure in the main

145

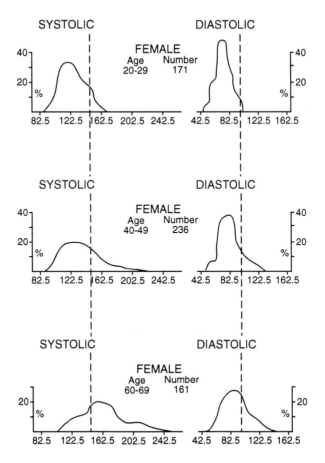

Figure 24 Frequency distribution of systolic and diastolic blood pressure in three groups of women, aged 20–29, 40–49 and 60–69. The curves were drawn by joining the percentage numbers of all cases in each individual group of people within a 10 mmHg range of blood pressure: e.g. 82.5–92.4 and 92.5–102.4 mmHg. The interrupted vertical lines mark off groups of women with blood pressures of 160/100 or more, i.e. definitely 'hypertensive'. Note that more women over 60 have systolic blood pressures greater than 160 mmHg than have systolic pressures less than 160 mmHg. (Drawn from individual data in a population study by Hamilton M et al., Clin Sci 1954; 13: 20).

(systemic) arteries goes up a lot, partly because hard muscles squeeze soft blood vessels. When the exercise stops, blood pressure goes back to normal. In established hypertension, on the other hand, blood pressure is consistently above normal even at rest.

146

Causes

There are many recognised specific causes of sustained hypertension. Kidney disease is the best understood and will be discussed in the next chapter. Since kidney disease can cause hypertension and hypertension can damage the kidneys we have the ingredients for a vicious circle. But the kidneys appear normal in young people with essential hypertension. None the less, many people believe that subtle changes in the way the kidneys operate can raise the blood pressure even though the kidneys look normal under the microscope. Nothing totally disproves this theory. There has also been a resurgence of interest in hypertension due to excessive production of blood-pressure-raising 'steroid' chemicals from the adrenal glands, especially aldosterone. Some people estimate that 5–10% of people with apparently 'essential' hypertension (see below) could be suffering from a subtle excess of aldosterone.

Despite this, for reasons which will become clear, I have found it intellectually more satisfying to propose a cause for essential hypertension which gives a primary role neither to the kidneys nor to the adrenal glands. Hypertension appearing towards the end of pregnancy is described in Chapter 17. Twelve causes of human hypertension due to a mutation in a single gene have been identified, but they are very rare. All such causes, together with kidney disorders, account for only some 10–20% of cases of established hypertension. The cause of the rest is unknown. Such people are described as having 'essential hypertension'. This antiquated term has stuck, but all it means is 'high blood pressure of unknown cause'. An essential hypertensive individual is defined as one whose blood pressure lies in the upper range of the normal distribution curve – above an (arbitrary) level of, say, 140/90 – and in whom no specific cause can be found.

Is there a real problem about 'the' cause of essential hypertension?

Sir George Pickering, a former Regius Professor of Medicine at Oxford, challenged the idea that there might be a specific cause for essential hypertension. He regarded it as simply a quantitative deviation from the norm and therefore thought that there was no point in looking for a specific single cause.

I shall illustrate the weakness of his argument by an analogy. Suppose that in the country of Erewhon the sphygmomanometer has not been invented, but that somehow doctors there have invented an instrument which when placed on the chest wall measures the resistance to blood flow in the coronary arteries of the heart. They call the measurement 'CVR'. Although they don't know exactly what they are measuring, their population surveys reveal skewed bell-shaped frequency/distribution curves of CVR looking just like those for blood pressure (Fig. 24). One of their Regius Professors says that there is no point in looking for 'the' cause of high CVR, because it is just 'a quantitative deviation from the norm', even though Erewhonians know that people with high CVR die young. But then one of their pathologists correlates measurements of CVR in life with post-mortem findings. He notes that people with high CVR have lumps of white material (atheroma) partly occluding the coronary arteries, whereas those with low CVR don't. So here is a highly specific condition, the severity of which is normally distributed in the adult community.

Instead of trying to find an all-or-none cause for essential hypertension let us postulate that its cause might be both well-defined and infinitely graded (as random arterial obstruction by atheroma clearly is).

High blood pressure and the nervous system

I have written two monographs suggesting that the brain initiates most cases of apparently 'essential' hypertension[1,2]. The word 'neurogenic' in the titles of these books implies that the hypertension is created by the nervous system. Many laymen, and some doctors, regard essential hypertension as a psychosomatic disease. In the USA particularly, the high prevalence of hypertension in blacks has been ascribed to suppressed hostility. Fear, anger and mental stress are well-known to raise blood pressure transiently. But there is no good evidence that strong emotions cause established essential hypertension. Psychological testing has failed to identify hypertensives in a population of young people who had no prior knowledge of their blood pressure. The strongest rebuttal came from the large trial organised by the British Medical Research Council[3]. Twelve thousand people filled in a well-validated questionnaire before their blood pressures were known. Later analysis failed to find any link between hypertension and potential psychological factors.

In the last 100 years huge advances have been made in many other fields, but the cause of essential hypertension remains elusive. There seem to be too many contenders rather than too few, as Fig. 1 (p. 2) shows. For fun, I calculated the exponential equation which describes this 'curve of discovery':

$$y = 1 + .05 (x - 1900) + .06 (0.05x - 95)^4$$

This suggests that a lot of presently unknown mechanisms controlling blood pressure have yet to be discovered. If the curve continues for another 100 years, we might expect another 500 new discoveries. This may sound ridiculous: but just wait!

The concentration and effective (partial) pressure of carbon dioxide (the waste gas produced by food combustion in the body) is closely regulated by the brain, by its control of breathing. Holding the breath raises carbon dioxide concentration; overbreathing reduces it. Increased concentration of carbon dioxide gas directly dilates blood vessels, but this effect is antagonised by increased sympathetic nervous activity. Curiously it has recently been found that the hormone insulin (deficiency of which causes diabetes) has actions which parallel those of carbon dioxide. Insulin itself is a vasodilator material, i.e. when infused into an artery supplying an organ or tissue it increases the local blood flow (by increasing the rate of production of nitric oxide). But it also acts directly on the brain to increase sympathetic nervous activity. This has a constrictor effect on blood vessels. As in the case of carbon dioxide, the two mechanisms cancel each other out. Insulin has almost no net effect of blood pressure when it is infused or injected. However, there is much interest in the possibility that changes either in insulin secretion or in the chemical receptors with which insulin combines might play a subtle part in causing high blood pressure, especially when high blood pressure is combined with obesity.

Alcohol in many circumstances raises blood pressure, possibly through an action on the brain; but people with essential hypertension can be lifelong teetotallers.

Genetic influences on blood pressure

Heredity is certainly an important factor. By comparing identical and non-identical twins it is possible to calculate to what extent someone's blood pressure is determined by heredity and how much by external environmental factors. The answer is about half and half. The genetic influence on blood pressure is 'polygenic', i.e. the result of the interaction of several genes. A large number of genes, each affecting one or more of the important blood pressure control factors shown in Fig. 1 (p. 2), might play a part. There is no single gene which on its own determines whether someone will or will not get essential hypertension.

There is some evidence, both in man and in animals, that the lower an individual's birth weight, the higher his or her blood pressure as a adult will be[4]. Dispute still rages over the meaning of these observations because of the multitude of possible confounding factors, especially the mother's blood pressure inheritance. But the blood pressure differences are anyway small and do not account for more than a small fraction of the wide variations in blood pressure between adults.

Genes influence the degree to which an individual's habitual intake of salt affects blood pressure. In susceptible people, the more salt they eat the higher their pressure. I shall return to this theme in the next chapter.

Negative feedback systems

A major problem in hypertension research is the large number of mechanisms stabilising blood pressure over time. Most of these utilise the 'negative feedback' principle. Blood pressure in the aorta and in the main arteries of the neck is continuously monitored by tiny sensors in the walls of large arteries, the arterial baroreceptors, described in Chapter 4 (see p. 32). If pressure rises, these send up to the brain via the vagus and glossopharyngeal nerves an increased electrical discharge frequency. The coordinating centres in the brain stem then send nerve messages to the small blood vessels in the body telling them to relax and lower blood pressure. The opposite happens if blood pressure falls. The brain then sends out nerve messages to constrict small arteries and veins to raise blood pressure again.

The kidneys provide another example of a blood pressure stabilising system working by negative feedback. If blood pressure rises, the kidneys excrete more salt and water. This reduces the amount of blood in the circulation and blood pressure goes down. If blood pressure falls, the kidneys hold on to fluid, thirst is increased, the volume of blood rises and pressure is restored.

There are several other known stabilising systems. All have one characteristic in common: they stabilise blood pressure over short periods of time but not over long ones. They reset their range of operation. It is as if the control system says: 'O.K., somebody, I don't know who, wants my blood pressure to go up from 120/80 to 200/120. As he insists on this I will have to permanently change my operating system. In future I will regard 200/120 as the pressure I need to maintain. I will keep it at that level, come what may'. So even if this hypertensive individual loses a pint or two of blood through an accident, blood pressure will be back almost to 200/120 in a few minutes. Retention of fluid will expand blood volume again in less than 24 hours, so that the brain will no longer need to send extra nerve impulses out to make arteries constrict.

To solve the mystery of essential hypertension, we need first to identify the basic master control system. Then we might be able to find why it is misbehaving.

Young inbred hypertensive rats can have their blood pressure kept low for many weeks or months by appropriate drug treatment. When treatment is stopped blood pressure may remain down. This does not seem to happen in man. In one big trial by the British Medical Research Council a large number of hypertensive people were treated for six years continuously with so-called hypotensive drugs. When treatment was stopped, to find out whether it was still needed, the blood pressure climbed quickly back to its original level six years before[5]. Evidently, therefore, people with essential hypertension have suffered some change which prevents the blood pressure being reset back to normal levels, even though pressure has been kept down for months or even years.

Where is the master controller?

This is where I get autobiographical and heretical. In 1958–9 I was a Research Fellow in the Middlesex Hospital Medical School in London. I attended the post-mortem room there and looked at the main brain arteries of nearly 100 people who had died in hospital and who were being examined to find the cause of their death. I had the idea that maybe the cause of essential hypertension lay in the brain, which raised blood pressure when it wasn't getting enough blood. But I must first explain the historical background.

Nearly 100 years ago Harvey Cushing, the famous American neurosurgeon, had observed that when the arterial blood supply to the head of a dog was restricted its blood pressure went up. This phenomenon is now known as the 'Cushing response'. Drawing on these observations, and on experiments of his own in the 1920s, Ernest Starling, the greatest English physiologist since William Harvey, suggested that essential hypertension might be due to 'gross lesions in the arterial trunks [which] might diminish the average pressure in the arteries of the brain. ... This condition is well known'. Two observations then came along to put this idea back on the shelf. First, fast-reacting baroreceptor nerve endings were discovered in the walls of the main arteries supplying the brain. When blood pressure in these arteries goes down, the change is detected by the baroreceptors and a signal is sent up to the brain. The brain then puts the blood pressure up again by a reflex action through the sympathetic nervous system. This discovery appeared to remove the need to invoke a contribution to the Cushing response by the brain itself. Second, in the 1940s, Seymour Kety devised a clever indirect method of measuring total cerebral blood flow (CBF) in awake man. CBF was found to be substantially normal in essential hypertension.

151

More recent work has shown that total brain blood flow is in fact somewhat reduced in essential hypertension, on average. But even if it had been found to be absolutely normal, I never felt that it was logical to argue that hypertensive individuals had nothing wrong with the blood supply to their brains. Could it not be that the rise in blood pressure was a response needed to keep CBF normal? Hypertension could then be regarded as an appropriate response to increased resistance to blood flow through the brain.

To test this hypothesis, Drew Thomson and I examined the large neck arteries (the internal carotids and the vertebrals) and the large cerebral arteries within the skull in our series of cadavers. The main arteries arise within the chest close to the heart, pass upwards along or within the neck bones, through the base of the skull, entering the brain as illustrated in Fig. 22 (p. 137). We thought that disease of these arteries might supply a substantial added resistance to the flow of blood to the brain. Fig. 25 (opposite) shows on the left X-rays of one fairly normal left internal carotid and vertebral artery in a woman of 43 whose blood pressure had been almost normal during life and on the right arteries from a woman of 59 with severe hypertension whose right internal carotid and (especially) vertebral artery is irregularly and grossly narrowed. In each case post-mortem artery spasm was first fully relaxed with ammonia. Then the same pressure of 140 mmHg of warm radio-opaque gelatin solution was applied to each artery (tied off at its ends) until the gelatin had set. X-rays were taken at the same standard tube distance in each case. Clearly there is very gross narrowing of both arteries in the hypertensive woman. The central channel (the 'lumen') of the vertebral artery, which supplies the hind brain is reduced almost to pinhole size. The internal carotid artery is larger but also considerably narrowed. Inspection of the arteries concerned showed that the narrowing had been caused by patchy deposits of 'atheroma' (Greek: ear of corn/porridge), a hard cheesy material mostly made up of cholesterol. It is obvious that extensive disease like this must have greatly increased the resistance to blood flow to the brain during life.

The technical difficulties of this type of study can easily be imagined. But since we were only interested in the resistance to the flow of blood through these arteries we decided for the whole series of cadavers just to measure the rate at which water could be forced through the neck arteries from their origin inside the chest to their termination inside the skull. This then avoided the need for dissection of the neck. We used a standard pressure of 140mmHg, after relaxing post-mortem spasm with ammonia. The results were very exciting. We found that there was a close inverse relationship between the fluid-carrying

152

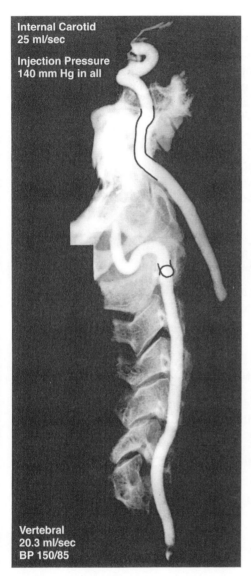
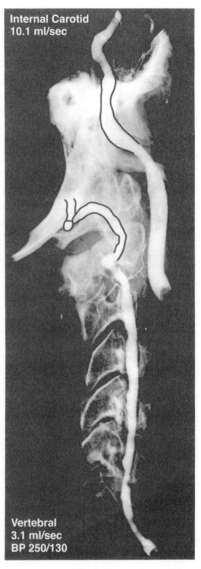

Figure 25 X-rays of the main brain arteries on one side of the neck in two human cadavers, showing the routes of the two arteries in relation to the bones of the neck (vertebrae) and the base of the skull. The vertebral arteries take a twisting looping course. A shows a normal vertebral and internal carotid artery in a 43 year-old woman with a near normal blood pressure. B is from a woman of 59 with severe hypertension and gross stenosis of both arteries by atheroma. The perfusion rates for each artery were measured as described in the text. Then a hot solution of gelatin containing X-ray opaque barium sulphate was pumped in and allowed to set while a pressure of 140 mmHg was maintained.

153

capacity of the arteries, especially of the vertebral arteries in the neck, and the blood pressure in life, which a kind friend (Jack Howell) got independently for us from the hospital notes (Fig. 26). An equally close correlation was also apparent between the blood pressure recorded during life and the number and extent of visible lumps (plaques) of atheroma in the vertebral and basilar arteries supplying the brain stem (Fig. 22, p. 137). This measurement was simple to make once the brain had been removed from the skull. Similar comparisons of kidney artery calibre at the time of post-mortem showed only a moderately close association with blood pressure during life. Similar measurements on the main leg (femoral) arteries showed almost no correlation between blood ante-mortem blood pressure and femoral artery fluid-carrying capacity.

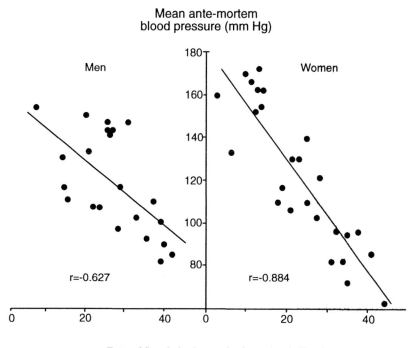

Figure 26 Correlation, in 22 male and 26 female cadavers, between the maximum rate of fluid flow in both vertebral arteries added together, at a standard pressure of 140 mmHg in all cases (as described in the text) and the mean blood pressure recorded in the hospital notes during life. The correlations for both men and women are highly significant. (Data from data of Dickinson CJ & Thomson AD, Clin Sci 1960; 19: 513–538).

Scientists recognise that correlations and associations, however close, prove nothing. All one can say is that if someone was looking for a cause of essential hypertension, narrowing of the arteries supplying blood to the hind brain would answer well. Although it is now generally accepted that narrowing of hind brain arteries is closely associated with essential hypertension, most people would conclude that high blood pressure has caused the arterial narrowing rather than the other way round. This view cannot be faulted since in several situations hypertension can be shown to increase the deposition of atheroma and thus potentially make arteries narrower.

Apologia pro vita sua

It is a strange and sometimes uncomfortable feeling to find oneself, as I do in respect of the cause of essential hypertension, holding views which almost no-one else accepts. But providing that scientists have not committed the capital scientific crime of falsifying or inventing data, they can be respected if not believed if they can stand by their ideas and defend them in argument. Often there is no universally accepted theory to explain a particular phenomenon. Several theories seem plausible. This then creates an intellectual battlefield in which each group of scientists supporting a particular theory competes with other groups supporting different theories. Each group tries to find logical flaws and contradictions in alternative theories. Such contests can be very exciting, though it is sad when emotional proponents of a disproved theory cannot accept defeat.

The close involvement of the nervous system in hypertension, especially in its initiation, is now better recognised than it was at the time of our post-mortem study. But as I mentioned earlier many people think that psychological factors are much more important than physical factors. And many of those who reject psychological theories of essential hypertension give pride of place to the kidneys rather than to the brain. Readers of my next chapter will realise that although the brain can certainly raise blood pressure in the short term by increased sympathetic nervous activity, hypertension can only be sustained if the kidneys collaborate. They certainly have the means to do so. The sympathetic nerve supply to the kidneys can cause constriction of their small arteries. Furthermore, the secretion of the hormone vasopressin by the posterior pituitary gland at the base of the brain controls water handling by the kidneys. Both brain and kidneys must be involved in sustaining hypertension, but dispute continues to reign over which is the prime mover.

Most current ideas about the cause of hypertension are centred mainly on the circulating chemicals which alter the calibre of blood vessels and on the receptor chemicals with which they interact. Many attempts have been made to link essential hypertension with genetic differences in some of these circulating chemicals and their receptors. During these investigations a number of specific single gene defects causing high blood pressure have been identified. But in the great majority of cases we still do not know what has gone wrong.

Animal models

In various centres, notably in Japan, the USA, New Zealand and Italy, attempts have been made to breed hypertensive rats so that the causes of high blood pressure could be better studied. By measuring the blood pressure of a group of rats and progressively mating the more hypertensive ones with each other various inbred strains of hypertensive rat have been produced. The best known was introduced more than 30 years ago in Japan by Aoki and Okamoto. It is internationally known by and assigned the name 'SHR', which stands for 'spontaneously hypertensive rat'. It was derived from a parent strain, the 'WKY' ('Wistar-Kyoto') rat, by selective inbreeding.

This rat strain has proved immensely useful for testing blood-pressure-lowering drugs. But I don't share the current universal enthusiasm for assuming that study of SHR tells us much reliably about the cause of human essential hypertension, even though grafting a kidney from an SHR can raise the blood pressure of a WKY rat, and replacing the kidneys of an SHR with a WKY kidney lowers blood pressure. This may tell us a lot about rat hypertension. Even though some comparable observations have been made in man, they do not necessarily prove anything about the initiation of essential hypertension. They do not prove that essential hypertension has its origin in the kidneys. Children with higher than average blood pressures tend to get higher than average blood pressures as adults, a phenomenon referred to as 'tracking'. But the effect is small. Essential hypertension usually starts to show itself in the third and fourth decades. Spontaneous hypertensive rats behave differently. The blood pressure of SHR begins to diverge substantially from that of WKY from the time of birth. There are many other differences. The strong current interest in the inbred hypertensive rat has skewed hypertension research very strongly away from man and towards the rat model. It seems to me more helpful to concentrate on the possible causes of blood pressure elevation in man which appear in the third and fourth decades.

None the less it is fascinating that although the brain arteries in the

SHR are not affected by atheroma, they are smaller than in the parent WKY strain. Consequently, tying off a main brain artery in an inbred stroke-prone hypertensive rat produces much more extensive damage to the brain than tying off the same artery in a rat with a normal blood pressure. This has made me speculate that just possibly the hypertension of the inbred hypertensive rat may have something to do with its inadequate brain blood supply, as I have envisaged might be going on in essential hypertension in man.

Why does drug treatment of hypertension protect against strokes?

One particular reason why my views about structural lesions of brain arteries underlying 'essential' hypertension are unacceptable to most people is that hypotensive (blood-pressure-lowering) treatment protects against strokes. This protection is well established. It is indeed the main reason for treating high blood pressure. The risk of strokes caused by arterial rupture and bleeding into the brain (cerebral haemorrhage) will obviously be less if the blood pressure is reduced by drugs. This is easy to understand. But the majority of strokes are not caused by bleeding but rather by cerebral 'infarction' (Latin: 'infartus' = something stuffed in). This is a technical term which means death of a tissue because of a critical reduction of local blood flow. It may be due to a local blood clot, or to an 'embolus' (Greek: 'patch' or 'something put in') – a clot formed elsewhere and swept in by the flowing blood. Although it seems paradoxical, drugs lowering blood pressure have been observed to protect spontaneously hypertensive rats against cerebral infarction.

The probable reason why lowering blood pressure can protect both rats and human beings against cerebral infarction is somewhat complicated. First, blood pressure can be reduced a lot before cerebral blood flow starts to fall at all. This is the property of the cerebral circulation known as 'autoregulation'. Therefore, moderate blood pressure reduction poses no immediate threat to the vitality of the brain. Second, blood pressure during 24 hours is very variable, especially in people with severe hypertension. Pressure can go up suddenly. Then arteries exposed to sudden peaks of high internal pressure may constrict. Arterial constriction has been directly observed in experimental animals with hypertension. If such arterial spasm continues after blood pressure has fallen, the stage would be set for a potentially critical reduction of blood flow to the affected area, causing cerebral infarction.

Conclusion

To do justice in a brief review to all current ideas about the cause or causes of high blood pressure is impossible. I have summarised my own heretical views in two books and in many published articles. They have been presented most fully in a recent monograph[2]. But someone wanting to explore in depth the better-established theories about this fascinating topic should consult a large multi-author review where all the vastly different views of different authors can be sampled[6].

Hypertension is an extremely common condition. It can be effectively treated by a bewildering array of different drugs. Drug companies are intensely interested in the cause of essential hypertension, in case its understanding will lead to better drugs being introduced. So it seems very unlikely that future research into this fascinating field will be curtailed by lack of money!

Summary

High blood pressure in the main arteries of the body is partly genetic, probably involving many genes. It is also partly environmental, being influenced especially by diet. Its main cause or causes are not known in most cases. It has a deleterious effect on health and lifespan, which are both reduced in proportion to any sustained elevation of blood pressure.

Many possible mechanisms are currently under investigation and the inbred hypertensive rat is the focus of much research. I doubt whether this animal is a good model. Essential hypertension in man does not usually show itself until the third or fourth decade and it is accompanied by arterial disease, especially of the brain circulation. We do not know at present whether the arterial disease is cause or effect. If it is cause, it probably operates through the 'Cushing' response, the control of which is located in the brain stem. Cerebral arterial atheroma provides a plausible structural basis for elevated basal blood pressure in hypertension.

This is only one theory among many. There is no agreement among investigators about the cause of essential hypertension, though there is growing recognition that the central nervous system plays an important role. The kidneys are also necessarily involved in sustaining hypertension of any cause. Many people believe that the kidneys are more likely than the brain to initiate essential hypertension, for reasons which will be examined in the next chapter. The disagreements and uncertainties reflect one of medicine's greatest current mysteries.

16

HYPERTENSION FROM THE KIDNEYS

In the last chapter I summarised what is known about so-called 'essential' hypertension – high blood pressure of unknown cause. Most known causes of hypertension involve the kidneys in some way. Indeed, many researchers believe that the kidney is the chief culprit even in essential hypertension, though this is hotly disputed. In this chapter I shall concentrate on those situations where sustained high blood pressure can reasonably be described as having a 'renal' (Latin: 'ren' = kidney) cause, even though the precise mechanisms involved may be disputed. Again I have to apologise for this chapter being somewhat autobiographical because I have been personally as interested in renal as in essential hypertension. But I will try to provide an unbiased account.

The functional anatomy of the kidneys

The two kidneys lie at the back of the upper abdomen on each side of the vertebral column. Each comprises approximately 1 million similar units known as 'nephrons' (Greek: 'nephros' = kidney). These are closely packed. Each nephron has a 'glomerulus' (Latin: from 'glomus' = ball, of yarn or wool), so named because it is a closely packed ball of capillaries. These make up a filter which holds back blood cells and protein molecules, but lets through water and small dissolved molecules such as glucose and urea, and metal ions like sodium and potassium. Each capsule which collects the glomerular filtrate leads to a convoluted tubule which joins up with tubules from other nephrons and eventually empties into the bladder. Vast quantities of blood pass through the kidneys each day (about 150 gallons) and similarly vast quantities of fluid are filtered out into the tubules (about 40 gallons). Almost all of this is reabsorbed back into the bloodstream, leaving a residue of urine of only 2–3 pints or so a day for an average fluid intake. The daily filtrate contains more than 2 pounds weight of salt (sodium chloride), but almost all this is also reabsorbed, together with the water. This leaves only about ½ ounce of salt to be excreted in the urine each day. Over long periods of time the urinary salt excretion is the same as the amount of salt in the diet, less the amount lost in sweat and other secretions.

The processes of salt and water reabsorption require energy. At rest about one fifth of the total energy consumption of the body is expended by the kidneys, mostly by the chemical processes actively reabsorbing salt from the glomerular filtrate. The whole process seems incredibly wasteful of energy, but it allows extremely flexible adjustments of kidney function to changes in diet and to intercurrent disease.

Kidney diseases raising the blood pressure

Richard Bright, a physician at Guy's Hospital in London, studied kidney disease. In 1836 he reported that some people suffering from kidney disease had a pulse which was 'full and hard'. When the sphygmomanometer was invented an association was quickly recognised between kidney disease and high blood pressure. Almost any kind of kidney disease can be associated with hypertension, but it is often difficult to prove causation. Most medical kidney diseases affect both organs. Both kidneys obviously cannot be removed to see whether they are causing hypertension, though a raised blood pressure can often be brought back to normal, for a time at least, by replacing diseased kidneys with a normal one.

Apart from renal artery narrowing, the commonest serious kidney diseases accompanied by high blood pressure are various forms of 'chronic glomerulonephritis'. In these conditions the delicate filters of the kidneys become inflamed, damaged, and eventually destroyed. When the kidney of someone in an active phase of glomerulonephritis is examined under the microscope (which can be done in life by taking a minute biopsy specimen with a needle) the filters of the kidney (the glomeruli) are thickened, inflammatory cells are abundant and the small arteries leading to the glomeruli are narrowed. Life can continue even if only 10% or even fewer kidney units are still working. Thus the greater parts of both kidneys have to be destroyed before there is any life-threatening failure to excrete the body's waste products. One clue to glomerulonephritis is 'proteinuria', the appearance of undue quantities of protein in the urine. This is caused by breaks in the glomerular basement membranes, i.e. in the filters themselves.

The end stage of chronic glomerulonephritis looks very much like the end stage of severe untreated essential hypertension. In both cases the failure of the excretory function of the kidneys can lead to death from renal excretory failure unless a kidney transplant can be done in time. Most patients with long-standing glomerulonephritis are hypertensive, sometimes even before there is substantial damage to the glomeruli.

The definitive animal experiments on renal hypertension were done by Harry Goldblatt. When I lived for a year in Cleveland, Ohio, I heard Goldblatt deliver his famous lecture describing how he came to create hypertension in dogs by interfering with the blood supply to their kidneys. He was a pathologist who had looked through the microscope at slices of kidneys from people who had died from complications of high blood pressure. He had observed that all the small arteries leading to the glomeruli were narrowed. Their muscular walls were thickened. He thought that perhaps constriction of the blood supply to the kidneys might have in some way caused high blood pressure. He wanted to imitate nature experimentally, but realised that he could not possibly put constricting clips on all the many thousands of minute arteries in each of the two kidneys. So he devised a marvellously ingenious but simple experiment. Under a general anaesthetic he exposed both kidneys of dogs, then put constricting clips across both main kidney arteries so that the blood flow would be reduced, but not actually cut off. (Cutting off all blood supply to the kidneys would obviously just make the kidneys die.) The blood pressure of dogs with constricting renal artery clips rose and stayed up. Goldblatt reckoned that he had got an exact model of sustained high blood pressure in man. Many people still agree with him and his experiments have been duplicated in many other species. Main renal artery stenosis (Greek: 'stenos' = narrow) is a well recognised cause of high blood pressure in man (see below).

Causes of renal hypertension

At least three renal mechanisms can raise the blood pressure. All appear to be simple, yet the more closely one looks at any of them the more complex they become. I shall describe them briefly under three headings:

1 failure to excrete enough salt and water;
2 overproduction of the blood pressure raising hormone 'renin';
3 failure to produce enough of a blood pressure lowering hormone, e.g. 'medulli(pi)n'.

Failure to excrete enough salt and water

Destruction of many nephrons by disease or by an impaired blood supply will obviously reduce the amount of blood filtered. But at the same time much less fluid and salt will be reabsorbed in the convoluted tubules because of a phenomenon called 'osmotic diuresis', caused by the high concentrations of dissolved materials in the blood and hence in the glomerular filtrate. This is the situation in the early stages of progressive kidney disease. The daily urine volume is substantially normal or even increased and in balance with fluid intake. Only in the later stages does the urine volume decrease.

If someone with renal excretory failure continues to drink and eat normally the body will start to accumulate water and salt after about 90% of all the nephrons have been lost and kidney function is down to 10% of normal. At this stage there may be what used to be called 'dropsy'. The medical term is 'oedema', i.e. swelling of the ankles which can be indented by gentle pressure, showing that there is fluid that can be moved about under the skin. However, tissue fluid is in a state of dynamic equilibrium with the blood in the circulation. If salt and water are retained in the body the volume of the blood also increases. By a process which is not fully understood even today this leads to a rise in blood pressure. A simple way of explaining what is happening is to look at Fig. 27, which shows what Jon Thompson and I observed when we perfused excised rabbit kidneys with blood at different pressures[1]. The higher the perfusion pressure the faster the excretion of water (and also of salt). In life, the curve is steeper still. It is easy to see how the body might compensate for failing to excrete salt and water by putting up the arterial blood pressure supplying the kidneys. This then allows the usual dietary intake of salt and water to be excreted and stability to be regained.

Severe renal excretory failure has to raise the blood pressure. If it didn't the body would swell up and harmful waste products would accumulate. The mystery is to explain how an increase in the volume of the blood raises the arterial blood pressure. The greatest living circulatory physiologist in the world (Arthur Guyton, in Mississippi) has always ascribed the hypertension of blood volume expansion to what he has called 'whole body autoregulation'. This is complicated to explain, but it follows old observations in Holland of the hypertension which can follow eating too much liquorice, which was in use at the time for the treatment of stomach ulcers. Liquorice contains a chemical which makes the kidneys retain salt and water. Guyton's arguments are set forth clearly in his books and articles[2]. Most people agree with him, though the curious involvement of the nervous system in this type of hypertension needs clarification. There is also evidence for at least two other entirely different mechanisms which can affect kidney function and affect salt and water excretion when the blood volume is expanded.

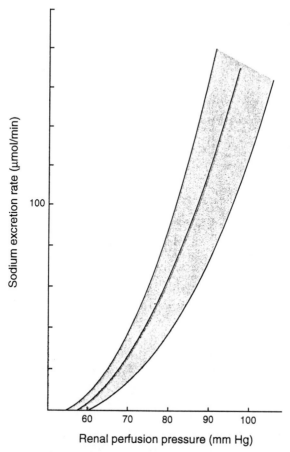

Figure 27 Mean results with 95% confidence limits obtained from 16 excised rabbit kidneys perfused with blood over a range of pressures, showing how the rate of excretion of sodium increases ever more rapidly as the pressure of blood perfusing the kidneys is increased. (Drawn from data of Thompson JMA & Dickinson CJ, Clin Sci Mol Med 1976; 50: 223–236).

Guyton's classic experiment is worth mentioning. In its simplicity and elegance it is a match for Goldblatt's renal artery clamps. Under general anaesthesia Guyton and his colleagues removed one kidney from a dog, and also cut out two thirds of the bulk of the remaining kidney. So long as the dog continued to drink water and to eat a normal diet it remained healthy, with a normal blood pressure. But when salt was added to the drinking water, and nothing else was changed, the blood pressure rapidly rose and remained high until the extra salt was withdrawn, after which blood pressure went back to normal.

Armed with the knowledge which this and comparable experiments provide, doctors treating advanced kidney disease pay great attention to their patients' intake of salt. It cannot be doubted that overload of the body with salt can cause hypertension, even though some of the details still need to be worked out. Curiously some people are sensitive to salt excess and easily get high blood pressure whereas others seem to be resistant. Similar differences have been noted in different strains of rat.

Although changes in blood volume in Guyton's experiment were undoubtedly the eventual cause of changes in blood pressure, the blood volume changes were obviously due to the extra salt. If the concentration of salt in the blood rises there is increased thirst. The posterior pituitary gland in the brain sends a chemical message to the kidneys to retain water until the concentration of salt is normal again. Thus salt and water go hand in hand, though water follows salt rather than the other way round. The medical treatment of excessive fluid accumulation, such as occurs with heart failure, usually involves giving drugs (diuretics) which make the kidneys excrete more salt.

Overproduction of renin

Adjacent to each outer glomerulus in each kidney is a tiny collection of cells known as the 'juxta-glomerular apparatus'. This is a ductless gland which secretes into the blood flowing through it two hormones. One is concerned with red blood cell formation. The other is importantly linked with blood pressure control. It is a protein called 'renin', which is an enzyme (a catalyst) which turns an inactive circulating material produced mainly in the liver (angiotensinogen), into a small polypeptide (angiotensin I) which is further changed by another (converting) enzyme into angiotensin II, one of the most powerful blood pressure raising agents known. There is an amusing story of the derivation of this hybrid name: two rival groups of people were working on the same material at the same time, one calling it 'angiotonin' and the other 'hypertensin'. They met at breakfast, split their differences, and created 'angiotensin'.

One way of making the kidney produce large amounts of renin is to restrict its blood supply (e.g. by putting a constricting 'Goldblatt' clip on the main renal artery). This sharply raises the blood pressure of any rat, rabbit or dog on which this has been done. I have seen the comparable experiment in nature when a blood clot detached itself from the heart wall of one of my patients and almost completely blocked one main kidney artery. As in the animal experiments, blood pressure rose rapidly and only went back to normal after the offending clot was removed.

Angiotensin II is a small polypeptide containing 8 amino acids. When infused into the bloodstream of any animal it constricts arteries and raises the blood pressure. This has been established in human volunteers as well as in animals. Fig. 28 is a personal record of the effects on blood pressure of infusing pure angiotensin II into a rabbit over a period of three days. The blood pressure rose to a plateau where it remained until the infusion was stopped.

Everything then seemed simple and straightforward. The hypertension caused by narrowing of the main kidney artery is a well recognised cause of maintained hypertension in man. It seemed reasonable to ascribe it to a circulating excess of renin and angiotensin. But there is a snag. Careful measurements of the amounts of renin or angiotensin in the blood of people with renal artery stenosis and hypertension showed that the amounts present did not seem to be enough to raise the blood pressure significantly.

While pondering this apparent anomaly I had the idea that maybe renin secretion was only switched on when the perfusion of blood through a kidney was reduced and that it was turned off again when blood pressure rose. Perhaps this might explain why there did not seem to be enough renin and angiotensin circulating. I therefore constructed an elaborate piece of hydroelectric equipment which continuously sampled a rabbit's blood pressure and which made the infusion rate of intravenous angiotensin inversely proportional to the animal's blood pressure at any moment. The effects were spectacular: it was just about the most exciting piece of research I have ever carried

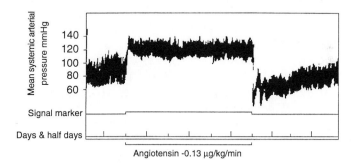

Angiotensin -0.13 µg/kg/min

Figure 28 A six-day record of the mean blood pressure of a rabbit, during which angiotensin was infused intravenously in high concentration for 3 days, as shown by the signal marker. The blood pressure went up rapidly by about 40 mmHg, remained steady for 3 days, then dropped immediately when the infusion was stopped. Damped oscillations with a 4-hour period continued as the blood pressure slowly returned to its control level over the ensuing 2 days.

165

out. Over a period of 2–3 days the delivery rate of angiotensin went steadily down at the same time that the blood pressure steadily rose. Later Jim Lawrence and I[3] found that it was simpler just to infuse angiotensin at a very low ('sub-pressor') rate, below that which initially produced any detectable rise of blood pressure (Fig. 29). Then Richard Yu and I found that these sub-pressor infusions of angiotensin had in some way activated the sympathetic nervous system[4]. I thought that this might be because angiotensin had constricted the brain arteries (as it is known to do). I tried to prove this by infusing angiotensin at very low rates directly into the arteries supplying the brain stem in rabbits. This also proved to be a spectacular experiment. It raised blood pressure tremendously, though not in the way I had anticipated. The experiment was serendipitous. The underlying hypothesis was mostly incorrect. The main effect of infusing angiotensin into the brain stem arteries was a direct neuronal stimulation of the brain centres controlling the sympathetic nervous system rather than an indirect effect mediated through arterial constriction[5].

Failure to produce enough of a blood pressure lowering hormone

Although salt and water overload and/or renin oversecretion explain most forms of renal hypertension, other observations show that the central part (medulla) of normal kidneys secrete a blood-pressure-lowering factor ('medullipin')[6]. Damage or removal of this part of the

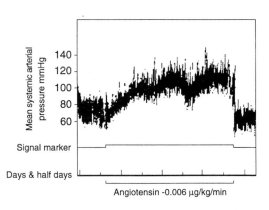

Figure 29 A 4–5 day record made in the same way as in Fig. 28 but showing the different effect of infusing a low concentration of angiotensin at a rate which had no immediate effect on blood pressure. The average blood pressure climbed up by about 35 mmHg over 3 days, but dropped sharply when the infusion was turned off[1].

166

kidney can raise blood pressure, and (rare) tumours secreting medul-lipin can show themselves by excessively lowering blood pressure. Lack of medullipin probably contributes to hypertension in many cases of renal disease.

Other mysteries of renal hypertension

Perhaps my explanations of those renal hypertensive mechanisms on which I have worked myself has made them seem unduly simple. Alas, this is not so. I have only given the barest outline of an enormous subject. For example, the cause of chronic glomerulonephritis has not been established for sure, though there is much evidence to suggest that it may be an auto-immune, perhaps an 'infective-immune' disease. A host of different materials – the steroid hormones and atrial natriuretic factor – affect salt handling by the kidneys and indirectly influence blood pressure. The well-known heart drug digoxin is now known to have close chemical and pharmacological similarities with a naturally occurring circulating material identical or almost identical with the plant derivative 'oubain'. This material affects kidney as well as heart function. The relationship between angiotensin and the central nervous system is only beginning to be explored, as we realise that angiotensin is itself an important neurotransmitter within the brain.

The way in which an animal gradually adapts to a blood-pressure-raising stimulus (such as the angiotensin infusion already described) involves many changes. Over long periods small arteries gradually get narrower, the heart muscle becomes thicker and many other changes occur which allow hypertension to be sustained with little evidence remaining of its initiating factor. These adaptive changes make it extre-mely difficult to decide which change is primary, and which secondary.

The study of renal hypertension has been of immense clinical value. The many animal experiments which have revealed the underlying mechanisms have resulted in the synthesis of angiotensin converting enzyme inhibitors (e.g. captopril) and of angiotensin antagonists (e.g. losartan), which are of enormous value in many conditions other than renal hypertension, e.g. heart failure and diabetes. The story continues to unfold. Plenty of mysteries remain to be solved.

Summary

Kidney disease, of which the commonest type is chronic glomerulo-nephritis, is often associated with high blood pressure. Three mechan-isms (at least) may be responsible:

1 renal excretory failure, especially of salt and water;
2 overproduction of renin and hence of angiotensin;
3 lack of production of medullipin, the renal medullary hormone.

Renal excretory failure expands the volume of circulating blood which leads to hypertension by a process which can be described as 'whole body autoregulation'. Although there may be very little renin circulating in many varieties of renal hypertension, renin generates angiotensin, a powerful hormone which raises blood pressure. Angiotensin exerts a slowly developing, partly neurogenic, action increasing over many days. In addition, the central part (medulla) of each kidney produces a blood pressure lowering factor, medullipin. Deficiency of this material may also play a part in producing 'renal' hypertension.

17

PRE-ECLAMPSIA: PREGNANCY-INDUCED HYPERTENSION

Pre-eclampsia (P-E) is a common and uniquely human disorder, although a somewhat similar condition has been reported in some patas monkeys. It occurs throughout the world, with an incidence, in different regions, of between 2% and 10% of first pregnancies. It is best regarded as a 'syndrome', i.e. a cluster of abnormalities. In a woman more than 20 weeks pregnant these are:

1 a rising blood pressure;
2 excessive amounts of protein in the urine;
3 (occasionally) swelling of the ankles due to fluid accumulation.

The protein in the urine suggests that the filters of the kidney are damaged and leaky. Although the term 'pre-eclampsia' is still in common use, it is a bit misleading, because actual 'eclampsia' is now extremely rare. That word comes from Greek, meaning a shining or violent bursting forth. This is not a bad description of the fits (convulsions) which characterise eclampsia. Good antenatal supervision can almost always prevent fits occurring. However, the term 'pre-eclampsia', meaning a step on the way to eclampsia, will doubtless continue to be used until the cause of the syndrome is discovered.

A woman whose mother or sister has had P-E is somewhat more likely to get it herself in her first pregnancy, so there is a significant genetic component. But a recent study of 471 female twin pairs failed to find even one in which the disease had occurred in both members. Lots of women get P-E without any family history of the condition. The pre-existence of a so-called 'collagen vascular disease' (such as systemic lupus erythematosus – see p. 74) makes the occurrence of P-E more likely, probably because the placental[*] blood supply may be impaired by the disease.

---

[*] The placenta (commonly known as the 'afterbirth') is a large plate-shaped fleshy structure which by the end of pregnancy is about 8 inches in diameter and weighs a bit

Towards the end of a first pregnancy, about one woman in 100, on average, will need to be admitted to hospital because of a diagnosis of P-E. She will be closely observed and probably have labour induced, or a Caesarian section carried out, within a week or two – usually because of rising blood pressure or signs of fetal distress appearing[*]. One in 200 women will require immediate termination of pregnancy for the sake of both mother and child. P-E can cause the death of a baby in the womb, or at the time of delivery. Maternal death in pregnancy is very rare, but eclampsia is an important cause of it. Eclampsia is not only characterised by fits but is also associated with damage to a mother's kidneys, liver, and her blood clotting system.

It is strange that a condition as serious as P-E doesn't usually make a pregnant woman feel ill. High blood pressure can cause headaches, but most commonly doesn't. Kidney damage produces no symptoms at all unless kidney function is very bad indeed. In days gone by, the occurrence of a fit was often the first sign that something was going wrong with the pregnancy. Nowadays prevention of P-E is the most important single aspect of care during pregnancy. Simple urine testing, taking the blood pressure, and checking for undue weight gain are the main needs. The modest costs of regularly checking these things is best regarded as insurance. Since P-E can appear with startling speed, current attempts to reduce costs by spacing out antenatal checks are misguided.

Since P-E is a uniquely human disorder it can only be studied in pregnant women. The ethical and practical difficulties of actual experiments are formidable. But we know how to cure P-E. The essence is to remove the placenta. Unfortunately a fetus is completely dependent on its placenta (Fig. 30). It will die in 15 minutes or so if the placenta is disconnected (e.g. if the umbilical cord joining fetus to placenta is cut or compressed). So cure of P-E has to involve removing the fetus as well as the placenta. If the baby is premature, experienced judgement is needed to say how long the pregnancy can be allowed to continue.

---

more than a pound. It is firmly attached to the inside wall of the womb (uterus) and connected to the 'fetus' (the technical name for a child still in the womb) by the umbilical cord). The placenta is a filter. It keeps back the mother's blood cells, and also most proteins, but it lets through water, glucose and other nutrients, and removes waste products. The filtered blood also supplies oxygen to the fetus and removes carbon dioxide.

[*] The main sign of the fetus being unwell is a fall in heart rate (below 110 beats/min), especially when accompanied by irregularity of rhythm. This usually reflects a poor placental blood supply and is what the midwife or doctor checks for with the ultrasonic fetal heart detector. An excessive rise of fetal heart rate (>170 beats/min) may also occur with fetal distress, but is uncommon.

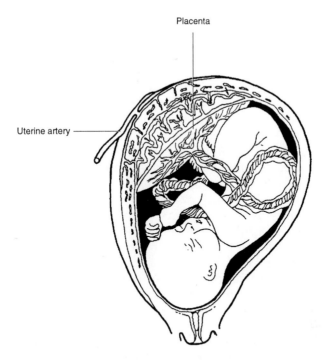

Placenta

Uterine artery

Figure 30 Diagram of fetus, placenta and uterus towards the end of pregnancy.

Usually two weeks is about the longest holding time when P-E is established because it almost never gets better on its own. Sometimes the concern in P-E is for the mother rather than the fetus, perhaps because of a disorder of maternal blood clotting or of liver function. But the usual worry is for the fetus.

Cause

The available evidence makes it almost certain that P-E is a primary malfunction of the placenta which somehow has bad effects on the mother. All the abnormalities of P-E disappear within a few hours or days after the placenta has been removed. The problems almost certainly involve the blood supply of the uterus and placenta. In P-E it seems as if cells derived from the fetus have failed to burrow well enough into the muscular wall of the womb to make adequate contact with the spiral uterine arteries coming from the mother to supply blood to the placenta. The mother's spiral arteries normally get larger as pregnancy progresses and lose their elastic and muscular coat, but

171

in some cases of P-E this function is defective. The immediate consequence is a restriction of the blood supply to the placenta and hence impaired transfer of nutrition to the fetus.

Lots of clues suggest that a placenta can set off P-E when it is not getting a good enough blood supply. This could be because the circulation of the womb is not fully developed in a first pregnancy, or because there is an extra load on the placenta (e.g. from having to supply blood to twins). Another possibility is that the placental circulation gets obstructed by blood clots. In P-E there is increased production of a chemical called thromboxane, which causes constriction of arteries and activates platelets – the tiny blood cells concerned in clotting. This suggested that aspirin, which reduces the stickiness of platelets and which gives some protection against coronary thrombosis might help to prevent P-E. So an enormous number of trials of aspirin have been made, but its benefits in P-E have not been convincingly established.

The placenta in P-E is commonly smaller than in a normal pregnancy and shows various types of damage, some of an inflammatory nature, some probably due to lack of blood supply and some due to local clot formation. Occasionally the placenta may appear normal on ordinary inspection. Secondary effects include a rise in the mother's blood pressure and a leak in her kidney filters, causing excretion of much more than the normal trace of protein.

A possible chemical factor?

It seems almost an inescapable conclusion that some chemical material produced by an 'ischaemic' placenta (one with an inadequate blood supply) passes into the mother's body and sets off the various changes. For many years many people have looked for some such material. Powerful hormones which are known to raise blood pressure (e.g. renin, angiotensin, noradrenaline and endothelin) have not so far been convincingly incriminated. There is some evidence of a deficiency of the blood pressure lowering material nitric oxide and a deficiency in the enzyme responsible for its synthesis. There may also be a slight deficiency of a hormone called 'adrenomedullin' (a polypeptide which also lowers blood pressure). We do not know the reason for these observations. None of the observed differences in circulating hormones or other factors so far examined can fully explain P-E.

There is recent evidence that blood serum taken from pre-eclamptic women increases the permeability to protein of endothelial cells lining blood vessels, whereas serum from normal pregnant women and even from women with pre-existent high blood pressure does not[1]. The particular interest of this last report is that the serum factor which causes excessive permeability of endothelium disappears within a few days of delivery, just as P-E does.

The authors of the report also produced some evidence that the factor might be an enzyme called protein kinase C which is an intermediate facilitator activating many cellular processes. However, protein kinase C is involved in so many activation processes in so many different cells that the general good health and well-being of most women with P-E is difficult to reconcile with the overproduction of some material involved with so many different actions. I would rather suspect that the excess of the enzyme is the result of a more fundamental pathological process.

Apart from the placenta secreting some directly damaging material into the maternal circulation, perhaps it can produce something which has an indirect effect (e.g. by acting on the brain or spinal cord). There is already evidence, from direct recording of sympathetic nerve impulses going to leg muscles, that the rise of blood pressure in P-E may be in part 'neurogenic', i.e. brought about by the nervous system. Perhaps the material presumed to be coming out of the placenta in P-E could be something which acts on the brain[2]. In that case one may ask whether a general increase of sympathetic nervous activity (SNA) can cause damage to endothelium and cause previously normal kidneys to leak protein into the urine. I think this is unlikely because when SNA is increased to the same or to a greater extent in essential hypertension we don't see endothelial damage or large amounts of protein in the urine. But perhaps increased SNA from the brain is due to some chemical from the placenta which causes damage to endothelium and leakage in the brain's blood vessels. Perhaps it is this leaked material which increases sympathetic nervous activity and puts the blood pressure up. This seems to me the most likely scenario.

Another suggestion is that there is overproduction of an endothelial 'suppressor factor', derived from a placenta poorly supplied with blood. A factor of this type, suppressing cell growth in tissue cultures, has been identified when endothelial cell cultures are treated with blood plasma derived from women with P-E[3].

There is some evidence that an inadequate blood supply to the placenta makes it produce an excess of certain cytokines – chemical substances such as 'tumour necrosis factor alpha' (TNFα) and 'interleukin-I' (IL-1). When these enter the mother's circulation it is envisaged that they damage the endothelial linings of her blood vessels. This structure seems to suffer the greatest damage in P-E. Instead of being smooth and reasonably watertight, the endothelium becomes unduly sticky and unduly leaky[4].

173

One might envisage that a placenta that is not working properly could make the fetus produce some damaging material which comes back through the placenta and enters the mother's circulation. For various reasons this is rather unlikely. There have been cases in which P-E has persisted after the baby has been delivered and has only been cured when a placenta still within the womb has been removed. Confirmation that the placenta is the villain of the piece also comes from examination of the placentas of pre-eclamptic pregnancies. They commonly show 'infarcts' – scars produced by lack of blood supply. Fortunately the fetus itself usually remains healthy providing that P-E is not allowed to get out of control. It is surprising that retarded fetal growth is uncommon.

Immunological aspects

So what on earth is going on? One suggestion is that the fetal part of the placenta, which necessarily has fetal rather than maternal genes in its cells, is acting as an antigen – a material which excites an immune reaction of some sort in the mother. Some cells circulating in a mother's blood can often be identified as having come from her fetus and have even been suspected of causing chronic disease in the mother (e.g. scleroderma). The mother's immune system certainly seems to be involved in P-E[5]. Exposure to chemicals derived from another individual and capable of producing an immune reaction (so-called 'foreign antigens') can eventually give a woman some protection against P-E even though at first they produce an adverse reaction. Previous blood transfusion from an unrelated donor has been observed to reduce the risk of P-E. A previous pregnancy will have exposed a mother to fetal antigens. This may explain why P-E is typically seen in first but not in later pregnancies. Yet another way appears to be the practice of oral sex without a condom. A long period of previous cohabitation with the same partner has been reported to give protection[6]. However, a second pregnancy with a new partner seems to bring a woman's risk of P-E back to what it was in her first pregnancy. Other observations by the same authors have suggested that conception within four months of cohabitation has a 50% chance of bringing about P-E in an ensuing (first) pregnancy, whereas after one year's cohabitation the chance of P-E drops to about 4%[7].

This extraordinary result certainly suggests that an immunological reaction, probably to a specific man's sperm in the vagina, may play some part in causing P-E. If so, protection against P-E may be provided by the woman's immune system becoming tolerant of a parti-

174

cular man's sperm. It reminds me of the best known example of immunological tolerance of foreign cells. This is the improved survival of kidney transplants in people who have previously had blood transfusions. If all these remarkable observations on P-E are correct (and some have been disputed) they could provide a plausible evolutionary advantage for a woman to stick to one partner while she is having children. Perhaps marriage can receive approval from scientists as well as moralists. One may even speculate historically that the institution of marriage itself might have evolved because it gave mothers-to-be the best chance of avoiding P-E.

A large recent study has reported that if a woman becomes pregnant by a man who has already fathered a pre-eclamptic pregnancy in a different woman, her risk of P-E is significantly increased[8]. It would therefore appear that paternal genes could play some part in causing the condition. The same survey also gave some limited support to the influence of cohabitation already mentioned[7]. Potential antigens in semen need to be itemised, to find whether there is for each a corresponding maternal antibody which increases during prolonged cohabitation with one man. Some really classy chemistry and immunology will be needed!

Though I am not an obstetrician and have never worked on P-E, it has always fascinated me. It is very common and of enormous social and economic importance. If I were now engaged in active research in P-E I should be examining placental extracts for their possible effects on the autonomic nervous system, i.e. those parts of the nervous system which are outside conscious control. If blood serum from women with P-E can be shown consistently and specifically to increase endothelial permeability in tissue culture outside the body, the way would be open gradually to focus down and identify the damaging chemical or chemicals. One would like to know whether the cells lining the blood vessels of the brain might be specially sensitive to placental extracts.

Another growing point of research is obviously going to be investigating placental factors controlling blood vessel growth in the later months of pregnancy. Failure of angiogenesis (growth of new blood vessels) evidently accompanies inadequate placental function, but whether this is a primary event impairing blood supply, or whether reduced blood supply impairs angiogenesis is debatable. Many different factors converge to stimulate production of 'vascular endothelial growth factor' (VEGF) (see p. 207). P-E might be due either to failure to produce enough VEGF or enough of one of its receptors. Some of the factors that might be involved are described in Chapter 21.

Summary

Pre-eclampsia (P-E) (pregnancy-induced hypertension with protein in the urine) is common, especially in the last three months of first or twin pregnancies. The mother may also develop swelling of the legs because of fluid retention. If the condition is left untreated it may result in death of the fetus and in extreme cases fits and even death of the mother. Prevention of P-E is the main purpose of antenatal supervision.

There seems no doubt that the immediate cause of the condition lies in the placenta. The condition usually resolves in a matter of hours after the placenta has been removed. The placenta usually shows scars of probable infarcts, suggesting impaired blood supply. One theory is that the fetal part of the placenta fails to make good enough contact with the maternal part, and that some material coming from the damaged placenta circulates in the mother, raising her blood pressure and damaging her kidneys. We do not know what this material is.

Much evidence suggests that there is some immunological intolerance by the mother's body of the fetus and its part of the placenta, and that this can set the syndrome off. This may explain why P-E is less common in second and later pregnancies.

18

PULMONARY HYPERTENSION

The normal pulmonary circulation

As I have already described in my introduction to Chapter 15, the lungs normally present little resistance to blood flowing through them. The pressures in the right side of the heart and in the pulmonary arteries are low (Fig. 23, p. 142). An adult lying flat, at rest, has a pressure in the main veins filling the right side of the heart of less than 3 inches (of blood: equivalent to about 5 mmHg). This is the height to which a column of blood would rise if it was connected to one of the great veins. The right ventricle of the heart pumps up the pressure to about 12 mmHg which drives blood through the lungs and into the left side of the heart. The powerful left ventricle of the heart pumps up the pressure to about 90 mmHg.

The pattern of blood flow through the lungs in someone standing upright is remarkable. At rest some 9 pints of blood (5 litres) flow through the lungs each minute. Virtually all the blood flows through the lower half of each lung. Almost none passes through the upper parts. Only during exercise, when the blood flow can increase up to about five times normal, does blood perfuse the upper parts of the lungs. This distribution of blood flow probably accounts for the location of secondary tuberculous infection at the top of the lungs (the apices) where blood flow is least. It also explains the benefit of supine bed rest which was cardinal therapy in the old tuberculosis sanatoria. Supine rest increases blood flow in the upper parts of the lungs. It probably gives the body's defences the best chance to resist the spread of infection.

One way of describing the normal pulmonary circulation is to say that it is like a waterfall. Once blood gets as far as the lungs of an upright subject it just tumbles through, with almost no resistance to its passage to the left side of the heart (Fig. 31). So although the lung blood vessels in a supine adult contains nearly 2 pints (900cc) of blood, during standing there may be only about half this amount. This explains why people whose heart is failing to pump blood adequately and who are breathless from lung congestion when they are lying

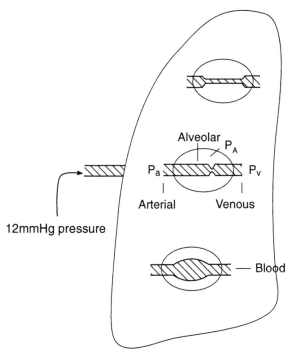

Figure 31 Diagram of three zones of the normal lung circulation in an upright subject. In the upper zone the surrounding pressure in the alveoli ($P_{\bar{A}}$) is greater than that in the lung capillaries ($P_{\bar{a}}$ to $P_{\bar{v}}$) which are pressed shut, so that little blood flows through the upper parts of the lungs. In the lowest zone the pressure in the pulmonary circulation is everywhere greater than the pressure in the airways and alveoli, so that blood flows freely through the lungs. Blood flow in the mid-zone fluctuates according to the phase of respiration. (Modified from an original diagram by Moran Campbell).

down get relief from standing or sitting. It also explains why blood letting ever became a recognised part of medical treatment. When shortness of breath is due to lung congestion, removal of blood can actually improve breathlessness. James Boswell, Samuel Johnson's biographer, records that Johnson obtained relief of breathlessness by being bled. However, in most situations blood letting is harmful. In times past it must often have supplied the *coup de grâce*.

Pulmonary hypertension

When, even at rest, the pressure of blood in the right ventricle and pulmonary arteries rises substantially above its normal 5 inches (12 mmHg) in a resting supine subject, the individual is said to have

178

'pulmonary hypertension', to distinguish it from high blood pressure in the rest of the body ('systemic hypertension'). An acceptable definition of pulmonary hypertension is a pulmonary artery pressure consistently at or greater than 25 mmHg at rest and 30 mmHg during exercise. From the description I have already given of the lung circulation it is obvious that pulmonary hypertension can only arise when more than half the pulmonary arteries are blocked, or when the average calibre of all the pulmonary blood vessels is reduced, or when the output of the right ventricle is twice as great as normal.

People with pulmonary hypertension get unduly short of breath during exercise and are sometimes breathless even at rest. Chest pain on exercise is often the first symptom. This probably arises because the heart muscle is not getting enough blood. Small arteries to exercising muscles dilate. If blood circulation is obstructed blood pressure falls.

Common causes of pulmonary hypertension

Sudden blockage of the pulmonary arteries will equally suddenly raise the pulmonary artery pressure. Pulmonary embolism describes a situation in which a blood clot, usually formed in the leg veins, passes up into the chest and along a pulmonary artery until it blocks it completely. If several large clots pass into both pulmonary arteries, the lungs will let very little blood through. The victim may die of 'shock' – a medical term which defines a potentially lethal reduction in the output of the heart. Pulmonary embolism is the most feared immediate complication of large surgical operations because of its suddenness and potential fatal consequences. Blood clotting in the legs is favoured by lying still for long periods. Not only surgical operations but also long plane journeys are potentially dangerous. People have to sit still, often cramped up. I have seen a previously fit young man who had travelled overnight from Hong Kong brought into hospital in London under my care almost at death's door, because of extensive pulmonary emboli. Fortunately it was possible to give immediate 'thrombolytic' injections of clot-dissolving material and save his life.

The consequences of pulmonary embolism seem easy to understand, but there is none the less a 'medical mystery'. Ventilation (the movement of air in and out of the tiny air sacs of the lung) is normally accurately matched to perfusion (the passage of blood through the walls of the air sacs). If ventilation is inadequate, as in asthma (see Chapter 2), the blood may not be properly oxygenated as it flows through the lungs. The patient may become blue. If the circulation becomes inadequate because of clots in the blood vessels one would expect such blood as did get through the lungs to be full of oxygen, especially because pulmonary embolism causes overbreathing (hyperventilation). Curiously, in pulmonary embolism the effects on oxygen supply are usually just the opposite. Too little oxygen in the blood ('hypoxaemia') is very characteristic of pulmonary embolism. The most likely reason is that some chemical factor or material produced by blood clots causes constriction of adjacent lung blood vessels. This could then disturb the normally good matching of ventilation and perfusion. It would be useful to find the cause of the mismatch, if only because the putative factor causing constriction of lung blood vessels might be related to the causes of longstanding 'primary' pulmonary hypertension (see below).

A more long-lasting obstruction to the lung circulation is provided by mitral stenosis. The mitral flap valve of the heart lies between the left atrium and the left ventricle. It prevents blood regurgitating from ventricle back to atrium when the ventricle contracts at each heart beat. Acute rheumatic fever, nowadays rather a rare condition, can damage the mitral valve and lead to its narrowing ('mitral stenosis'). Pressure then rises in the left atrium. This increases the pressure in the lung blood vessels and pulmonary artery. The right ventricle has to pump harder. The diagnosis is made by measuring the pressures at different parts of the system (using fine catheters passed up the arteries from an artery in an arm or leg). The defective valve can either by repaired or replaced. There is not usually any long-lasting lung damage if the condition is recognised in time. The pressures all go back to normal.

Widespread lung disease of any cause may make it difficult for blood to pass freely through the lungs. Some degree of pulmonary hypertension is common in severe chronic bronchitis with lung destruction and fibrosis. However, this is usually the least of the patient's problems, which arise from the lung disease itself rather than from any consequential circulatory embarrassment.

But there is another mechanical cause of pulmonary hypertension which has much more serious consequences. There can be a defect in the heart and blood vessels which lets some of the high pressure blood from the left ventricle or its outflow tract (the aorta) flow directly into the lower pressure right side of the heart. The defect usually arises during fetal life. It is therefore by definition congenital, i.e. something you are born with. There may be an atrial septal defect (ASD), a ventricular septal defect (VSD), a patent ductus arteriosus or sometimes even more complex mis-arrangements of the blood vessels or heart chambers. Small leaks of blood from left to right through one of these holes in the heart are of little consequence, but large leaks can cause serious trouble. The heart has to do much more work, since the blood transferred back from left to right side has to be pumped round again. At rest the total output of the left ventricle may be twice normal or even more. It is as if someone apparently resting had a lung circulation more appropriate to brisk walking. The pressure in the right ventricle and pulmonary arteries obviously has to rise once all the spare capacity of the pulmonary circulation is exhausted. Some people with substantial left to right shunts of this sort live reasonably normal lives, though with some restriction of strenuous sustained muscular exertion. Unfortunately in other cases – we don't know which ones will do this – changes gradually take place in the pulmonary circulation and start an inexorable and fatal vicious circle.

When this situation is recognised early, at birth, there is an urgent need to correct the defect, despite all the difficulties and dangers of large operations on tiny babies. Unfortunately after the structural changes in the lung circulation have taken place, correction of the shunt will not bring back normal conditions. Indeed, once the pressures in the right side of the heart rise to levels similar to those in the left side no shunting of blood will occur. An operation to close the hole in the heart becomes pointless, and may do more harm than good.

Primary pulmonary hypertension

Some unfortunate adults develop 'primary' or 'idiopathic' pulmonary hypertension, meaning pulmonary hypertension of unknown cause, when none of the mechanisms already discussed seem to be in operation. It is often associated with pulmonary 'fibrosis' (too much fibrous tissue in the lungs) which is often called 'cryptogenic fibrosing alveolitis'. ('Cryptogenic' means of concealed or of unknown cause; 'alveolitis' means inflammation of the very small terminal air sacs of the lungs, the alveoli). The condition is about twice as common in women as in men. It usually appears in early adult life at an average age for diagnosis of 35. It affects between one and two people per million of the general population. If it is not treated, or cannot be treated, average survival is only two to three years.

In some cases widespread small clots seem to be the underlying cause, sometimes associated with a recognisable disorder of blood clotting. In most cases, however, the small lung arteries just seem to get narrower, even though every other body system seems to be working correctly. Any long-standing elevation of pressure in the pulmonary circulation can eventually cause thickening of small arteries (arterioles) because of increase in muscle and fibrous tissue. There is also reduced synthesis of the dilating materials nitric oxide and prostacyclin and increased secretion of the constricting material endothelin-1[1]. Over-use of the appetite suppressors fenfluramine or aminorex has a definite association with pulmonary hypertension and may increase incidence as much as tenfold. These drugs are believed to act by increasing the local concentrations of serotonin (a blood vessel constrictor material). Several other drugs, especially anti-cancer drugs, have also been occasionally incriminated. Cigarette smoke has a small but measurable ill effect, increasing blood flow resistance in the lungs.

Most cases are sporadic and no cause can be discovered, though 6% run in families. Linkage of inherited cases to a gene on chromosome 2 at 2q31–32 location has been confirmed[2]. The immediate cause of the condition is an increase in bulk of the inner lining of capillaries and an increase in the bulk of muscle surrounding the small lung arteries. Several different patterns of disease have been recognised. The common feature is that the lungs develop increased resistance to blood flowing through them.

The vicious circle

A vicious circle may come into operation in any of the situations I have described in which the pressure in the right heart and pulmonary arteries is continuously well above normal. Established pulmonary hypertension is a very serious and intractable condition for which no fully effective treatment has yet been devised. Most people with a sustained pulmonary artery pressure of 3½ feet of blood (50 mmHg) or greater die within five years. It seems that a substantial rise of pulmonary arterial pressure stretches the walls of the smaller pulmonary arteries (arterioles); this supplies a stimulus for their muscular walls to constrict and eventually stiffen; the narrowed blood vessels increase the resistance to flow; and pulmonary hypertension becomes established and ultimately irreversible. Blood clots then often form in the small lung arterioles. This can increase flow resistance still more. Long-term treatment with anti-coagulant drugs such as warfarin improves prognosis in most types of pulmonary hypertension though it does not cure the condition. Reduced availability of oxygen tends to constrict pulmonary arteries, a reaction which has been observed in people living at high altitude.

There is an interesting contrast between systemic hypertension (Chapter 15) and pulmonary hypertension. Lots of drugs are known to lower blood pressure in the rest of the body. They do this by relaxing the muscular walls of the small arteries and are in widespread use for treating established systemic hypertension (see Chapter 16). They undoubtedly relieve symptoms and prolong life. Unfortunately none of them seems to have much effect on the small arteries of the lungs, at least when the dose is kept below that which would cause total collapse of the circulation. Lots of things have been tried. One of the most interesting is the gas nitric oxide, which is known to cause systemic arteries to dilate. It can be administered by inhalation. Some limited success has been reported, especially in children and the newborn. Unfortunately its effects seem to be rather short-lived. Many other dilating drugs such as hydralazine and nifedipine have been tried, but without well-established benefit. At the present time, epoprostenol (prostacyclin, a chemical produced by the body having a powerful short-term dilating effect on lung arteries) seems to be the most effective treatment, but it has to be administered continuously by infusing it slowly into a vein. Agents interfering with blood clotting are usually also prescribed, to reduce further damage by local small clots. In some of the worst cases lung transplantation seems to offer the only hope of survival. Some improvement in long-term survival can be obtained by mechanical means, surgically creating or opening up a hole between the right and left atria. This lowers pressure in the right side of the heart and in the pulmonary artery. Even though this lets venous blood containing little oxygen mix with oxygenated arterial blood, the result may be beneficial overall.

Cause

The site of increased resistance in sustained pulmonary hypertension is the small arteries (arterioles), but there does not seem to be any specially notable structural defect. It is just that the endothelium and muscle are thickened. It has been suggested that the matrix material surrounding small lung arteries may be abnormal and in some way affect muscular contraction of vessel walls.

If we knew everything about the control of the circulation through the lungs, we might be able to design a drug which would make more blood vessels in the lungs grow or open up more widely. There are local chemicals secreted by cancer cells which help to secure for themselves an adequate blood supply by opening up local blood vessels. I shall discuss this topic further in Chapter 21. Unfortunately no suitable factor with an action on pulmonary arteries has yet been discovered, though extracts from rapidly growing tumours are being tested by infusing them into the pulmonary circulation, to see whether they reduce pulmonary artery pressure.

If I were in the business of designing such a factor I would take a good look at chemicals derived from the gut. My reason for suggesting this will become apparent to those who have read Chapter 7. I summarised there the evidence that the normal liver probably inactivates or destroys some material in the blood coming to it which opens up lung blood vessels. Scarring of the liver (cirrhosis) is often associated with short circuits of blood passing through it and is sometimes also associated with clubbing of the fingers, probably because unmodified blood from the venous side of the circulation gets through to the main systemic side. Patients with severe liver disease have sometimes even been thought to have some form of congenital heart disease, because they had signs (undue blueness) suggesting a substantial shunt of blood from the right to the left side of the heart.

My guess is that the normal liver removes some substance or substances which are capable of opening up small lung arteries. Such material is most likely to be derived from the gut, or possibly from the pancreas. I have not the slightest idea what such a substance might be. Apart from the spleen and pancreas, the gut is the only large abdominal organ whose effluent blood drains through the liver. (Blood from the kidneys, for example, drains directly into the large veins taking it to the right side of the heart.) So it might be interesting to try various gut and pancreatic extracts to examine their possible effects on the lung blood vessels. Although pulmonary hypertension is fortunately rare, it is one of the most distressing conditions because of its relentless progress once a vicious circle has begun.

Summary

The normal pressure in the pulmonary circulation is low. The circulation there behaves as if it was a waterfall, with almost no resistance to blood flowing through the lungs.

Many conditions can raise the pressure (e.g. congenital heart defects with an abnormal communication between left and right sides of the heart; clots forming in or getting stuck in the pulmonary arteries; extensive lung disease with scarring). The most serious situation arises when the condition has been both severe and persistent enough to start off a vicious circle, which can reach an irreversible stage. At this point, treatment is difficult. Cadaveric lung transplantation may be needed. Continuous intravenous infusion of prostacyclin is the only moderately effective drug treatment. Some help may be given by surgically creating an atrial septal defect.

Evidence (summarised in Chapter 7) that some material coming from the gut or pancreas may dilate the lung circulation when it passes unchanged through the liver suggests the possibility that such a material might alleviate chronic pulmonary hypertension, a condition which has so far defied effective, convenient and acceptable treatment.

18

VASCULITIS: TEMPORAL ARTERITIS AND ALLIED CONDITIONS

The term 'vasculitis' is a diminutive of 'vas' = vessel, duct or pipe conveying fluid; and '-itis' = inflammation. The group of vasculitic disorders, collectively referred to as 'vasculitides', are rare conditions in which there is inflammation of the walls of blood vessels, especially arteries, leading to consequent ill effects on the organs or tissues involved. There is local inflammation and death of cells (necrosis), which take on an appearance known technically as 'fibrinoid necrosis'. There may also be 'granulomas' (the more correct Greek plural is 'granulomata'). These are microscopic well-circumscribed areas, firmer than the surrounding tissue. They contain characteristic large single-nucleus cells, sometimes with a few large cells with several nuclei ('giant cells'). Vasculitis may occur (rarely) in rheumatoid arthritis (see Chapter 8) and in other allied conditions; but I shall confine my discussion in this chapter to a few of the best known vasculitides. In all of these, inflammation of blood vessels is the predominant disorder.

Polyarteritis nodosa

When the larger muscular arteries are involved the condition is known as 'polyarteritis nodosa' (PN), that is, many ('poly') arteries with inflammation ('itis'), and with lumps or nodes ('nodosa'). Smaller arteries and veins can also be affected in an inflammatory process, which often involves the kidneys severely, sometimes leading to kidney failure. A large number of differently named sub-groups with some common features have been recognised, with exotic names such as Takayasu's arteritis, Henoch-Schönlein purpura, Behçet's disease, Churg-Strauss syndrome and Kawasaki disease. One of the commonest is temporal arteritis (see below). Any of the larger arteries, including the aorta itself, may be affected. Other rather similar conditions predominantly affecting small arteries include Wegener's granulomatosis, Goodpasture's syndrome, microscopic polyangiitis (hypersensitivity angiitis) and cerebral vasculitis. Fig. 32 illustrates the overlapping of the features of some of these conditions.

Most of them produce fever, aching in muscles and in joints, together with general feelings of tiredness and weakness. In most cases there is widespread involvement of many different organs and tissues. Blood markers of inflammation such as the 'ESR' (erythrocyte sedimentation rate) and 'CRP' (C-reactive protein concentration) are usually increased. Despite the similarity of these various conditions when the inflamed vessel walls are examined under the microscope, their natural histories are distinctly different. Many international conferences have attempted classification of these overlapping syndromes. I shall not attempt one of my own, but simply describe the main features of two common conditions and two rare ones which make an intriguing contrast with PN.

Temporal arteritis

I have looked after many people with temporal arteritis (TA). It typically affects elderly people. The first symptom may be a general

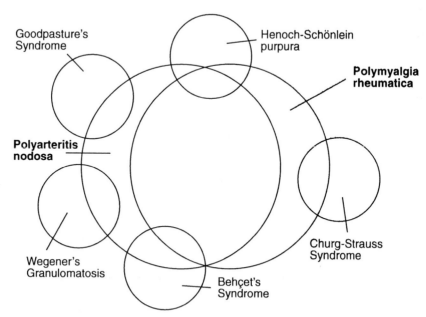

Figure 32 Diagram emphasising the overlap between various vasculitic disorders, affecting blood vessels of different sizes.

feeling of tiredness, with a low-grade fever, headache and weight loss. In classic cases there may also be tender points or actual lumps over the temporal arteries, which run across the outside of the skull across the temple, above the ear. For people over 50 the incidence of the disease is about 20 per 100,000 per year, though there are wide variations in time and place. The disease is about twice as common in women as in men. Though the temporal arteries themselves are not invariably affected and tender enlarged temporal arteries can be felt in less than 50% of patients, the diagnosis is usually and conveniently made by removing a tiny piece of a temporal artery and examining it under the microscope. (The temporal arteries lie only just beneath the skin, so that surgical access is easy; furthermore the blood supply of the scalp is so good that temporal artery biopsy is a harmless procedure when competently performed.)

Many physicians who suspect temporal arteritis will start patients on steroid drugs such as prednisone as soon as they suspect the disease, sometimes without even doing a temporal artery biopsy, because of the danger of sudden obstruction of the main eye (retinal) artery. This can lead to permanent blindness in the affected eye. I have never felt certain whether steroid drugs simply suppress the manifestations of the disease and allow it to disappear of its own accord, or whether steroids play a part in its eventual cure. The complications of temporal arteritis are due to obstruction of small arteries, especially those in the kidneys, but symptoms may arise from impaired blood supply to many tissues, including those of the brain, gut and other organs.

Polymyalgia rheumatica

Another condition – polymyalgia rheumatica (PR) – (from 'poly-' = many; 'my-' = muscle; 'algi-' = pain) affects a similar age group. It is also associated with the same changes in the blood, aching muscles, fever, and weight loss as are found in TA. PR is nearly twice as common as TA. Many people regard them as fundamentally the same condition. There are epidemiological parallels because the incidence of both diseases tends to rise and fall at the same time.

Acute infections often seem to be able to trigger TA. In the long run, TA usually gets better on its own, as does PR; but I have looked after patients who have required steroid drugs (usually oral prednisone) for many years to keep the diseases suppressed. One of my patients with PR had to take steroids for three years and one with TA needed treatment for five years. Both patients were eventually able to stop steroids when their pain and fever remitted and their blood tests returned to normal.

Henoch-Schönlein purpura

Henoch-Schönlein purpura (HSP) is one of the most interesting small vessel vasculitides. It causes a characteristic skin rash and joint pains. It may also involve the gut, causing colicky abdominal pain. Although there is often both protein and blood in the urine, kidney damage is usually mild and does not progress. It is commonest in childhood, but can occur at any age. There is a characteristic deposition of particular immunoglobulin E (IgE) immune complexes (antigen/antibody combinations) in many organs. The disease is unusual in that in most cases cure is spontaneous and occurs after the disease has run a course lasting only a few weeks. I have seen two cases, both in elderly men. It is very difficult to imagine that such a disease is not triggered by some infection arriving suddenly from an external source. It often follows an upper respiratory tract infection. It is highly likely that there is an as yet unidentified organism, which might be a virus or a bacterium, which sets off or triggers the auto-immune reaction which we recognise as HSP. The relative rareness of the condition makes it difficult to study. It can be confused with more serious conditions such as microscopic polyangiitis.

A patient may suffer from rather general symptoms before the diagnosis of HSP can be firmly made. This is a pity because the way in which it runs a self-limiting short sharp course in most cases might give us important information about the cause of commoner and more serious vasculitides.

Wegener's granulomatosis

Wegener's granulomatosis (WG) is much rarer than TA and usually begins at an earlier age, sometimes in childhood. The sexes are equally affected. The condition usually appears to start in the upper respiratory tract (that is, the nose and internal nasal passages), sometimes with ulceration and bleeding, together with many of the less specific features of TA. Later the lungs usually become involved, producing cough, chest pain and shortness of breath. The kidneys also eventually become involved in most (untreated) cases. Death from kidney failure is sometimes only preventable by a kidney transplant or by intensive immunosuppressive chemotherapy. However, with current treatment, combining the immunosuppressive drug cyclophosphamide with a glucocorticoid steroid (prednisone), the majority of patients achieve a remission, though relapse is common and may necessitate further courses of treatment.

The definitive tissue diagnosis is usually made by examining a small piece of tissue from one of the nose ulcers under the microscope. Certain changes in the blood – the appearance of antineutrophil cytoplasmic antibodies (ANCAs) – are particularly characteristic, though they may also occur in some rarer but rather similar conditions. 'Antineutrophil antibodies' are proteins, produced by lymphatic tissue, which attack and kill 'neutrophils'. These are blood cells called 'neutral' because they do not take up stains from certain dyes. 'Cytoplasmic' means 'pertaining to the cell body rather than to the nucleus'. In WG these antibodies attack some of the body's own defensive white blood cells by combining with a particular enzyme (proteinase-3) which is expressed on white cell surfaces[1]. So-called 'immune complexes' are formed by the combination of the circulating antibodies with complement (see p. 73) and with particular component parts of the white cells.

Cause

Only three causes of vasculitides such as PN, TA and WG seem likely and are currently being seriously investigated. They are:

1 An infection, which might involve:
   a) viruses;
   b) bacteria;
   c) fungi; and
   d) other larger organisms.
2 An immunological disorder, in which the body has become sensitised to some antigen (a material which triggers a response by the body's immunological system: see p. 27). Such an antigen could be:
   a) extrinsic to the body (e.g. ingested, inhaled, put on the skin);
   b) intrinsic, i.e. a normal body constituent to which the body has become sensitised, or which has been changed by a somatic mutation.
3 A combination of (1) and (2), in which an infection has precipitated an immunological disorder, either by the organism itself acting as an antigen, or by facilitating access to the body by a damaging antigen, or by changing the antigenic properties of some previously normal cells or tissues in such a way that they become antigens.

Almost all the available evidence favours involvement of the body's immune system in some respect in these conditions, if only because immunosuppressive measures and immunosuppressive drugs make these conditions better, even though they do not cure them.

Since ANCAs are so characteristic of WG, we need to consider what could have caused production of these apparently damaging antibodies. One possibility is that the disease has been started by an infection, perhaps by an (as yet) unrecognised bacterium, one of whose cell components is chemically similar to some material in normal white blood cells, perhaps the enzyme 'proteinase-3'. Then when the bacteria are detected by the body's immunological defences, antibodies are produced which destroy normal defensive white blood cells as well as neutralising the (presumed) infection. The fact that no infection has so far been identified means nothing. In the past there have been many infections which went unrecognised for years. *Helicobacter jejuni*, a main cause of peptic ulcers, is a good example.

In many respects these conditions resemble rheumatoid arthritis (RA) (see Chapter 8), but there are several notable differences which point to a different underlying cause. Whereas RA typically occurs in children and young adults, TA is almost confined to the elderly. It is rare under the age of 50, but becomes commoner with each later decade. Arteritis is not usually seen in RA, so that the most dreaded complication of temporal arteritis (blindness) does not occur.

It is very difficult to escape the suspicion that PN, TA and PR are triggered by an infection which induces a harmful immunological reaction in one of the ways I have envisaged. In the case of TA or PR the disease usually begins suddenly, within a week or two. It eventually burns itself out after months or years. If it had been induced by a somatic mutation, for example, eventual spontaneous cure would not be expected. Unfortunately we have no idea what might be the nature of the infection, nor why it should largely confine its attacks to the elderly. There has been some evidence to incriminate a triggering infection by various organisms, notably *Mycoplasma pneumoniae*. There has also been some suggestive evidence that *Parvovirus 19*, *Chlamydia pneumoniae* or Q fever might be involved. So far observations have been inconsistent. No known trigger factor can account for all cases.

WG is equally mysterious. Like TA it usually starts suddenly, but the indications of a triggering infection are considerably stronger. There is the way it usually starts in the nose, suggesting an airborne infection. In addition, the bacterium *Staphylococcus aureus* is found to be living in the nose of some 60% of people with WG. (This bacterium causes boils on the skin and infections elsewhere, but it can live in the nose cavity without necessarily causing any symptoms.) Not all patients with WG carry the organism. Only a few patients carrying the staphylococcus in their nose develop WG, though carriers are more prone to relapses than non-carriers. Thirdly, early cases of WG respond well to the combination broad spectrum antibiotic, trimethoprim/sulfamethoxazole. Finally, even though such treatment may eliminate the staphylococci from the nose, relapses of WG do occur. Indeed, complete cure of WG is exceptionally rare. This makes me wonder if some other, as yet unknown infective agent not only triggers WG but also perhaps makes it easier for the staphylococcus bacterium to live in the nose. Alternatively, a local staphylococcal infection in the nose might make it easier for some other infective organism to gain a hold.

A painful and unpleasant skin condition known as pyoderma gangrenosum may occur together with WG, as well as with many other inflammatory conditions of uncertain origin, such as inflammatory bowel disease: (p. 123). The association gives a further clue to the possibility of a hitherto unidentified infecting organism being involved in WG. It is interesting that dapsone and clofazimine (anti-bacterial drugs mainly used to treat leprosy) appear to be helpful in pyoderma gangrenosum in addition to standard treatment with immunosuppressive drugs such as steroids, cyclophosphamide and cyclosporine.

I cannot finish my account of WG without telling a bizarre but true story. When I was a junior doctor (a 'house physician' or 'intern') in 1953, my chief was Max Rosenheim, who was later elected president of the Royal College of Physicians. He had in his charge a middle-aged woman who was running a fever and who had a bloodstained discharge from her nose. Max made a clinical diagnosis of WG, which was confirmed by biopsy of an ulcer in the nose. At that time there was no treatment known to help WG. The diagnosis was equivalent to a death warrant. The kidney failure to which it appeared to be progressing was uniformly fatal. I therefore asked my chief if I could try some experimental treatment. On the assumption that a bizarre infection might be the cause of the disease I administered a full course of an organic antimony preparation (a rather toxic drug which was used to treat certain tropical parasitic infections, notably leishmaniasis). In addition I gave her a full course of potassium iodide (because at the time it had a reputation as an anti-fungal agent). To my chief's amazement, and mine, the fever went down and the patient made a full recovery, with no relapse. Everyone assumed that the diagnosis had to have been mistaken, that the patient (an ex-nurse) had been falsifying her temperature readings and that the nasal ulceration was caused by self-induced trauma – despite the firm diagnosis made by our pathologists on the basis of the nasal biopsy. But I have often wondered since this case if some very unusual organism might underlie WG and whether my choice of unconventional therapy might perhaps have cured the patient. Some extremely indolent forms of leishmaniasis are known. As far as I can discover no investigations of antibodies to leishmaniasis or other tropical diseases have been reported in WG.

It would be interesting to make a controlled trial of this therapy; but since combined immunosuppressive treatment usually controls the disease fairly well, even though it does not cure it, such a trial might be difficult ethically to justify nowadays. It is obviously a generally accepted rule that once any treatment has been shown to improve or control an otherwise fatal condition, it becomes unethical either to withhold that treatment or to administer a dangerous untested alternative.

Summary

There are many varieties of vasculitis (inflammation of blood vessels), which may affect large or small arteries and to a lesser extent, veins. Temporal arteritis (TA) and polymyalgia rheumatica (PR) are the commonest conditions. Each runs a course of a few years before resolving, usually spontaneously. Henoch-Schönlein purpura (HSP) may run a serious explosive course, but in most cases gets better on its own within a few weeks. Polyarteritis nodosa (PN) and Wegener's granulomatosis (WG) are more serious conditions which do not usually resolve spontaneously. They produce extensive systemic symptoms and organ damage, and usually require continuing immunosuppressive therapy.

In none of the 'vasculitides' I have discussed is the cause known, but many appear to be initiated by an infection in a genetically predisposed individual. They all involve the immune system and respond in various degrees to immunosuppressive drugs.

20

FOLIC ACID AND NEURAL TUBE DEFECTS

The body's need for vitamins

Vitamins are simple chemicals in our diet which the human body cannot make for itself, but small amounts of which are essential for life and health. Most are found in vegetables or fruit, some in other animals. Folic acid is not a natural compound; but when it enters the body it is converted to the natural vitamin tetrahydrofolate, which is required for all cell divisions and cell renewals. Adequate amounts are specially necessary in pregnancy. Folate is a member of the 'vitamin B_2 complex' family and has in the past been known as vitamin B_{10} or B_{11}. Its name comes from Latin ('folium' = leaf) because it is found particularly in green vegetables. Deficiencies of some vitamins cause well-recognised diseases, for example:

B_1: beri-beri
B_6: pellagra
B_{12}: pernicious anaemia
C: scurvy
D: rickets and osteomalacia

No named 'disease' has so far been linked with folate deficiency, though in adults lack of folate may cause neuropsychiatric disorders which resemble the neurological complications of vitamin B_{12} deficiency (see below). These may be relieved, even 'spectacularly', by the administration of 5–10mg of folic acid daily[1]. A low concentration of folate in the blood appears to increase the risk of premature atheromatous arterial disease, probably through its association with abnormally raised blood concentrations of the amino acid homocysteine. This is recognised as an important causal link to arterial disease. Fig. 33 illustrates in outline one of the chemical interrelationships which keeps the concentration of homocysteine low. The vitamin B_{12}-requiring enzyme (catalyst) methionine synthetase links folate supply with homocysteine metabolism. Lack of a supply of folate causes a build-up of homocysteine because its conversion into methionine is

195

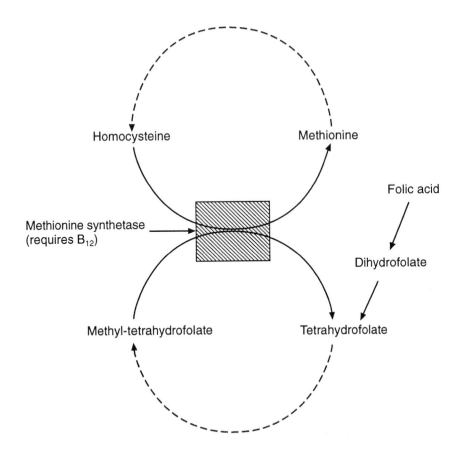

Figure 33 Diagram of one of the main chemical pathways which interrelate the chemical (metabolic) pathways by which the body keeps the concentration of homocysteine low by converting it into methionine. This is only possible if there is an adequate supply of folate and also of vitamin B_{12} (necessary for the action of methionine synthetase).

impaired. There are other chemical reactions involving the B vitamin pyridoxine (vitamin B_6) as well as folate, which also act to prevent a harmful rise in the blood concentration of homocysteine.

Tetrahydrofolate is necessary for many chemical reactions, particularly those involved with the synthesis of the building blocks of DNA. Folate deficiency interferes with the formation of blood cells. It can also damage the inner lining (endothelium) of blood vessels.

Folic acid-like drugs are used in the therapy of some malignant diseases. Thus folic acid could theoretically antagonise and potentially interfere with anti-cancer drugs like methotrexate which may themselves work in part by interfering with folic acid metabolism, but there has been little to suggest that this is a significant or serious problem. Although folic acid has in the past been thought to accelerate malignant change, the opposite is more likely to be the case. Animal studies have shown a protective effect of folic acid against some cancers[2]. In pregnancy there is some evidence that folic acid administration reduces the risk of premature births. It may also reduce or prevent other developmental disorders such as cleft palate and certain brain tumours in children. But the most important effect of folic acid is the protection it gives against neural tube defects.

Folate protects against nervous system maldevelopment and disease

The spinal cord is a slim (about ½ inch diameter) cord of nerve cells and nerve fibres, running from the back of the brain to the middle of the back. It is normally protected from injury by being enclosed by bony arches protruding from each of the vertebral bodies which make up the spine. During development the two sides of each vertebral arch close, thus forming the 'neural tube' which protects the delicate spinal cord within it. But sometimes development is incomplete. The vertebral arches do not close properly. This may allow the spinal cord coverings, or the delicate cord itself, to protrude out of the lower back, a condition described as a 'myelocele' (Greek: 'myelo-' = marrow; 'kele' = hernia). Many different severities of this condition can occur. All run the risk of damage to the spinal cord. This can cause a lifelong stiff paralysis of both legs (spastic paraplegia) or worse defects.

In the huge multi-centre British Medical Research Council trial a daily supplement of 4mg folic acid by mouth, before and during pregnancy, reduced by two thirds the risk of a woman having an affected baby[3]. The risk is even substantially reduced for a woman taking a supplement of only 0.4mg folic acid daily throughout pregnancy, compared with one taking no supplement. Other vitamins make no significant difference. We do not know for sure whether all mothers-to-be need extra folic acid before and during pregnancy. Concentrations of folate in red cells of the blood have been found to be less in women who have had children with neural tube defects than in a matched control group with normal children. Folate levels were lowest in women who had three or four affected offspring.

One important factor predisposing to neural tube defects may be an inherited disorder of folate metabolism causing a fault in body chemistry which is virtually the same as that seen in actual folate deficiency. This could explain why many mothers of neural tube defective children have blood folate levels well within the accepted normal range. The concept of a metabolic block has received further support from a comparison of dietary intake and folate levels between mothers of normal children and mothers of children with neural tube defects[4]. There may also be an increased rate of folate breakdown in the body in pregnancy and a consequential extra need for folate.

Clearly all women should take folic acid supplements before and during pregnancy. Under most circumstances 0.4mg daily is probably enough, but it is possible that more than this (i.e. 4 or 5mg daily) might be better, to overcome a possible metabolic block.

The possible bad effects of folic acid

The blood disease called pernicious anaemia (PA) was recognised around 1900. This is now known to be due to a failure to absorb vitamin B_{12} from the diet, usually because of stomach disease. The description 'pernicious' was given because, in addition to anaemia, patients developed unpleasant and ultimately fatal neurological complications (see below). Around the 1930s folic acid was found usually to correct or prevent the anaemia of vitamin B_{12} deficiency when taken by mouth. Unfortunately it was later found not to prevent the neurological complications. This was particularly unfortunate because folic acid is active by mouth, whereas B_{12} has to be given by injection.

We now recognise that giving folic acid to a patient with B_{12} deficiency can mask underlying disease and allow neurological deterioration. This should not happen if doctors are properly educated to check (by a simple blood test) for vitamin B_{12} deficiency in any person complaining of leg weakness, unsteadiness of gait, or of feelings of numbness or 'pins and needles' in the legs. Anaemia should not be regarded as a necessary accompanying sign of the neurological disorder.

Is folic acid a neurological poison for people with B_{12} deficiency?

Normal individuals have never been harmed by taking extra folic acid, even in a large dose such as 20 mg daily. But folic acid has a bad reputation in PA because of the suspicion that it is harmful when vitamin B_{12} is deficient. In the days before B_{12} treatment was introduced, PA patients who did not die of anaemia often succumbed to the unpleasant neurological condition known as 'subacute combined degeneration of the spinal cord'. The speed of neurological deterioration was extremely variable.

Unfortunately there were some reports of rapid neurological deterioration during administration of folic acid as sole therapy. Such experiences led to an important editorial in 1947 in the *New England Journal of Medicine* (probably the world's most influential medical journal) warning that an 'explosive onset' of neurological symptoms had been seen in many cases of PA treated with folic acid alone. The editorial stated that 'whereas although subacute combined system disease may start acutely, it does so rarely'.

Sometimes strong clinical impressions unsupported by rigorous statistical analysis become accepted truth. As a student I was taught that folic acid damaged people with B_{12} deficiency. This view is still widely accepted today. But it is always worth questioning accepted truth. The issue is important because of its relevance to food fortification. So I made a library search of clinical studies of PA published before 1930, before the introduction of either folic acid or vitamin B_{12}. These revealed that neurological deterioration was often quite as rapid and severe in otherwise untreated patients not given folic acid as in those given the vitamin, once it became available in the 1940s.

In situations like this animal evidence can be helpful. Large fruit-eating bats can be made deficient in vitamin B_{12} by manipulating their diet, whereupon they develop serious neurological deterioration and eventually die. There has been some evidence – indeed the only animal evidence we have (apart from a very small dog study) – that giving B_{12}-deficient fruit bats folic acid hastens neurological deterioration. I examined the evidence carefully and was unconvinced, for reasons which I have published elsewhere[5]. The big question remains: does folic acid cause or accelerate neurological damage to humans with B_{12} deficiency? There has never been a controlled, let alone a double-blind, comparison between the rate of neurological deterioration in PA with and without folic acid.

Theoretically, folic acid could act in various ways[6]. The most obvious is that it might reduce plasma B_{12} concentrations and hence accelerate neurological damage. There is no good evidence for this. Folic acid might have a direct effect on vitamin B_{12} metabolism, but no evidence has been found for this either. The relation between vitamin B_{12} and folic acid is complex. The cause of the neurological disturbances in vitamin B_{12} deficiency is not yet known. It may involve some as yet unidentified vitamin B_{12}-dependent enzyme. The speed of progression of neurological symptoms and signs in untreated PA is extremely variable. It can be rapid, with notable deterioration occurring over a few weeks. In the many published reports from 1947 onwards on folic acid being given to people with PA, I could find no evidence that the speed of neurological deterioration had been any faster than in untreated cases. In all the reports, serious neurological deterioration in PA patients treated with folic acid as sole therapy took between six weeks and 24 months to develop.

Subacute combined degeneration of the spinal cord is an alarming and unpleasant condition. It is not surprising that a doctor watching a patient over a few months become incoordinated, spastic, and unable to walk would describe the deterioration as 'explosive', perhaps not appreciating how rapidly progressive the untreated condition can be. Since giving vitamin B_{12} produces a complete cure of PA, whereas folic acid does not, it is now impossible (ethically) to compare the rates of neurological deterioration in untreated PA with PA treated with folic acid alone. But the proposition I arrived at by research in the library – that folic acid even in full dose (e.g. 4 or 5 mg daily) will neither cause nor accelerate neurological deterioration in pernicious anaemia – is not refuted by any solid published evidence. Likewise, it is not reliably contradicted by the only available animal evidence. I conclude that folic acid is intrinsically safe.

The case for food fortification with folic acid

Folic acid can be added to flour for making bread and pasta. It does not deteriorate during baking. Fortification of flour would ensure that most women would have enough folic acid in their bodies to protect against having a damaged spastic child. Many pregnancies, even as many as 50%, are unplanned and unexpected. Not all parents are both responsible and fully informed about the importance of folic acid supplements. Thus a very strong case can be made for fortifying flour with folic acid[7], especially since the need for the vitamin is greatest in the first few weeks of a pregnancy. However, bread in the shops is eaten by everyone. Some elderly people with PA will undoubtedly have their anaemic symptoms suppressed by folic acid, even by a small dose. How serious is this risk?

The pros and cons of food fortification

Having reviewed the evidence I suggest that the risk of doctors failing to diagnose PA early enough is now negligible. All doctors recognise the need for checking blood B_{12} concentrations in anyone with unexplained neurological symptoms or signs. The test is simple and cheap. The hypothetical side effects of flour fortification with folic acid have to be balanced against the certain benefit of preventing neural tube defects in unplanned pregnancies. I suggest that the case for universal fortification of bread and other cereals is thus very strong. The American Center for Disease Control Working Group recently calculated that if one third of a milligram of folic acid was added to each 100 grams of cereal grain, only 5% of the population would receive more than 1 mg daily of folic acid. This modest dose, which should prevent between 25% and 50% of neural tube defects, will almost certainly also prevent patients with vitamin B_{12} deficiency from becoming anaemic. But surely it will soon seem absurd that doctors need to see their patients becoming anaemic before they can make the diagnosis of vitamin B_{12} deficiency. As I have mentioned earlier, folic acid deficiency is suspected of causing mental deterioration, serious neurological symptoms and developmental abnormalities. It is therefore likely, though yet unproven, that some elderly people will be spared neuropsychiatric and other disorders if their usual diet contains extra folic acid. I have already mentioned that folic acid supplements lower the level of homocysteine and may thus also protect against arterial disease.

The possibility of inadvertently improving anaemia with big doses of folic acid in someone with vitamin B_{12} deficiency during pregnancy is small, because PA usually arises after the menopause. Furthermore, vitamin B_{12}-deficient women are often, though not always, sterile. Inadvertent folic acid administration may occur when multivitamin preparations are given and continued despite the appearance of neurological symptoms. Doctors need to bear this possibility in mind because many people take extra vitamins without consulting their doctors. Some anti-epilepsy drugs can cause an anaemia which gets better with folic acid. So if an epileptic person was in an early stage of developing PA and received added folic acid, the neurological symptoms of B_{12} deficiency could be masked. This seems only a theoretical risk. Anti-convulsants are prescribed by doctors who should be aware of this possible problem. They should therefore check the plasma vitamin B_{12} concentration in all suspicious cases.

As long as doctors are properly educated to have blood vitamin B_{12} concentration measured on everyone presenting with pins and needles or other odd sensations in the legs, unsteadiness, or unexplained limb weakness, no harm will ensue, though the situation will need careful monitoring. Most doctors are anyway aware that vitamin B_{12} deficiency is a common cause of odd neurological symptoms in people over 35 and that there is a high prevalence of borderline or actual vitamin B_{12} deficiency in the elderly. Neuropsychiatric symptoms have been observed in nearly a third of people with subnormal B_{12} levels, even though many were not anaemic. It seems to me that to withhold folate fortification of food because patients with PA may then not be ill enough for doctors to make a diagnosis promptly is absurd. It is as absurd as would be stopping the routine administration of iron tablets to pregnant women, for fear that the occasional case of polyposis coli[*] might be overlooked. Even as long ago as 1951, probably as a result of improved general nutrition, patients with PA were beginning to present themselves more often than before with neurological rather than anaemic symptoms.

How to proceed?

Although I believe that the current prejudice against universal folic acid fortification of food is based on anecdotal and scientifically invalid evidence and that the benefits outweigh the risks, a compromise of some sort may be needed. I hope that universal folic acid fortification of cereal grain may soon come about. Careful observation and recording of possible ill effects in the elderly should be combined with recording of what I anticipate will be beneficial effects: protection against neuropsychiatric, arterial and malignant disease. I have been an examiner in general medicine in many medical schools in Great Britain and abroad and can testify that most clinical students know that the neurological signs and symptoms of B_{12} deficiency may occur without anaemia.

We still do not know exactly how folic acid works, nor do we know why lack of vitamin B_{12} damages the nervous system. When these mysteries are solved it may become easier for everyone to accept the desirability of folic acid fortification of flour and to overcome the widespread natural prejudice against food fortification, even with a natural vitamin.

Summary

If an expectant mother takes a modest supplement of folic acid (one of the B_2-complex vitamins) before and during pregnancy she will prevent at least two thirds of the expected number of neural tube defects in her child. Folic acid also protects against a number of neuropsychiatric conditions in the elderly and may give some protection against coronary arterial disease.

Unfortunately it does not prevent the neurological complications of vitamin B_{12} deficiency, although it does prevent and correct the

[*] A rare but very dangerous pre-malignant condition of the colon which often comes to light by causing anaemia.

202

anaemia. Although folic acid is believed by some people to aggravate or even cause the serious neurological complications of vitamin B_{12} deficiency this fear is probably unfounded. The case for universal fortification of cereal grain with folic acid now appears to be extremely strong.

21

THE BLOOD SUPPLY OF TUMOURS

Sixteen years ago I wrote in '*The Encyclopaedia of Medical Ignorance*' that the way in which tumours got themselves a blood supply was a notable area of ignorance[1]. It still is, but vast strides have been made in our understanding. I have included this chapter because the subject is at the forefront of current cancer research. It has implications for many other normal and disease processes (e.g. fetal growth and wound healing).

Cancer starts when a cell in the body has suffered a sequence of 'somatic mutations' (see below), sometimes augmented by damage to genes involved in DNA repair or by a mutation in the tumour-suppressor protein (p53) which controls the programmed self-destruction (apoptosis: see p. 75) of abnormal cells. A propensity to cancer is often contributed by inherited DNA abnormalities. This means that a cell may start off already part way towards cancer. For example, the BrCa genes make breast cancer more likely in women who inherit them. (Two are known already, but clues from family breast cancer pedigrees suggest that several more await identification.)

The number of cell divisions of most body cells is limited because a bit of the end of each chromosome – the 'telomere' (Greek: telos = end; meros = part) – is lost with each successive cell division, until the cell dies. Normally about 200 units of DNA (technically 'base pairs') are lost from the ends of each chromosome at each cell division. Since there are several thousands of redundant non-functional 6-unit DNA sequences at the end of each chromosome, many replications are possible before cell function is compromised. But eventually, after perhaps 50 cell divisions, the cell loses vital genes and dies. We have known for many years that some cancer cell lines grown in culture in the test tube are immortal. They can continue to divide indefinitely without losing genetic material. The reason is the presence in nearly 90% of cancer cells of an enzyme called 'telomerase'. (This is technically a DNA polymerase, composed of ribose nucleic acid and protein sub-units.) This reconstructs the truncated or damaged ends of each chromosome each time the cell divides. The process may not necessarily be concerned in the initiation of cancer but is highly relevant for its later disastrous growth and spread around the body. Cancer cells can also become immortal by recruiting yet another mechanism for repairing chromosome ends, the 'alternative lengthening telomeres' (ALT) system.

A mutation can be defined as a change in some part of the DNA contained in a chromosome in the cell nucleus. A 'somatic' mutation means one pertaining to the body (Latin: 'soma' = body), i.e. one which develops after fertilisation of the egg. A skin papilloma is the consequence of a somatic mutation. Such a lesion tends very slowly to get bigger, but almost never disappears spontaneously. If one of its cells develops one or more further somatic mutations the tumour might become a so-called 'rodent ulcer', which is a localised form of skin cancer. This can get progressively bigger but does not spread from the skin into internal organs. To spread through the bloodstream (the most efficient way for cancer cells to spread to other organs) cancer cells need to degrade the matrix around a small blood or lymph vessel by secreting enzymes which digest proteins and fibrous tissue. This lets cancer cells into the blood flowing through the vein. Cancer cells may do this directly, or indirectly by stimulating normal large scavenger cells ('macrophages') to produce the necessary enzymes. In either case a certain minimum bulk of tumour tissue is needed.

But the mystery I want to discuss is not why a cell escapes from its normal controls and starts dividing, but rather how it manages to build up a mass of tumour tissue. How does it get itself a blood supply? All cells require a supply of food and oxygen to provide energy. If the main artery supplying a tumour is tied off the tumour shrivels up and dies. A malignant tumour – one which has lost all control over its cells dividing – cannot grow to more than about one tenth of an inch (2mm) in diameter unless it gets new blood vessels to supply its component cells with nutrients. The reason is the time it takes for materials to diffuse through the jelly-like material between cells. I have calculated the time it would take for 50% of molecules (individual chemical particles) to move various distances by diffusion alone through a stationary fluid, rather than by convection. Dissolved particles have to get through the walls of blood vessels, so the estimates of diffusion rates of glucose and protein molecules that I made in a previous chapter (see Table, p. 97) are certainly overestimates of the speed of diffusion. Although diffusion is extremely rapid across short distances it is very slow across large distances. (This is, of course, why all except the tiniest of animals and plants have developed some form of fluid circulation to allow nutrients to be brought to tissues and waste products to be removed.)

Angiogenesis (Greek: 'angio-' = vessel; 'genesis' = creation) has been described as driven by a cocktail of growth factors and pro-angiogenic cytokines and tempered by an equally diverse group of inhibitors of neovascularisation. Some 20 blood vessel growth stimulators and inhibitors are known, including 'epidermal growth factor' (EGF), 'platelet-derived growth factor' (PDGF) (p. 63), 'fibroblast growth factor-1' (FGF) and 'transforming growth factor-beta' (TGFβ). Most of these cytokines, possibly all of them, work by facilitating the production of one of the 'vascular endothelial growth factor' (VEGF) family which vary in their permeability and chemical properties. The basic molecule of VEGF closely resembles that of PDGF. Both are technically 'dimers', i.e. paired molecules. They combine with parts of the receptor chemicals which stimulate cell synthetic functions. Nitric oxide seems also to be needed. The main receptors are known as VEGFR1 (Flt-1) and VEGFR2 (Flk-1 or KDR) for VEGF, and the beta receptor for PDGF. There are natural stimuli which switch on or increase production of all these substances. Increased metabolic rate, which increases oxygen consumption and lowers its availability, is much the most important. Increased metabolic rate also increases the activity of another growth factor distinct from VEGF, angiopoietin-1, which stimulates growth when it combines with a receptor called Tie2, also known as TEK. The latter is located particularly in the thin lining membrane (the endothelium)[2]. Fig. 34 illustrates the relation between some of the main angiogenic factors. All this sounds complicated enough, but any idea that the whole story is nearing completion should be dispelled by current estimates that there are about 20,000 discretely different protein sub-units in each cell of the body.

The normal rate of division of the endothelial cells lining blood vessels is about one division every six months, but under appropriate stimulation in rapidly growing tumours the replication rate can be at least 50, possibly 500 times faster. The relevance of endothelial growth stimulators to tumour growth is attested by observations that a high rate of VEGF production in breast cancers is associated with a shorter survival.

Current interest in angiogenesis is growing because it opens up the possibility of inhibiting growth or spread of tumours by interfering with their blood supply. This might be done in many ways. The most obvious is to prepare an antibody to VEGF. Alternatively, VEGF might be linked to a toxin (e.g. diphtheria toxin[3]), thus producing damage to any cells which have receptors for VEGF. It might also be possible to prepare a chemical similar to VEGF but which would block its receptor. There are many possibilities. The main problem

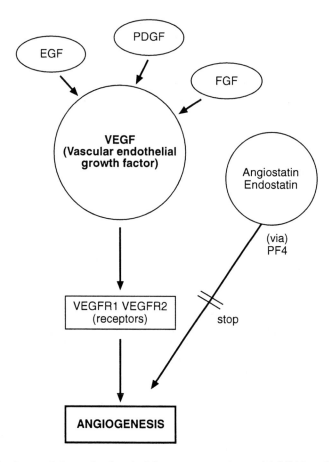

Figure 34 Some of the main chemical factors promoting and inhibiting the growth of blood vessels: EGF = epithelial growth factor; PDGF = platelet-derived growth factor; FGF = fibroblast growth factor; VEGFR1&2 = vascular endothelial growth factor receptors; PF4 = an angiogenesis inhibitor.

with this approach is that the processes of angiogenesis are also involved in wound healing, so that side-effects might limit this form of therapy. However, its use has already been envisaged for the treatment of tumours which are known to have a large blood supply.

New blood vessels can also be inhibited by naturally occurring anti-angiogenic (usually called 'angiostatic') factors such as angio-poietin-2, a naturally occurring antagonist for the Tie2 receptor. There is a particular family of related cytokines, the 'CXC chemo-kines', which can be either stimulators (e.g. IL-8) or inhibitors (e.g.

PF4) of angiogenesis, depending on whether or not one end of the molecule contains a specific sequence of three amino acids (see p. 85). Two further potent inhibitory factors have been identified by Judah Folkman's research group in Boston. (Folkman has been a leader since 1970 in the search for inhibitors of cancer angiogenesis.) 'Angiostatin' is a powerful inhibitor of the growth of endothelial cells. It has turned out to be a fragment of plasminogen, a naturally occurring protein present in blood plasma, which is part of the system of interacting chemicals in the blood which dissolves clots.

The action of angiostatin was noted in a most interesting way. A single large cancerous tumour growing in a mouse seemed to inhibit the growth of smaller tumours round about the main tumour mass. The responsible chemical was purified and then identified, after immensely painstaking work extending over many years[4]. The same group of investigators have more recently discovered an even more powerful inhibitor of blood vessel growth, 'endostatin'. This is part of the structural protein collagen XVIII which is found exclusively in blood vessels. It is present in detectable amounts in human circulating blood. A particularly exciting feature of endostatin function is that not only is it effective in shrinking malignant tumours in mice, it does not seem to induce resistance to its anti-tumour effects, as all standard anti-tumour drugs do. A recent report of the combined use of angiostatin and endostatin produced banner headlines in national newspapers because of the spectacular inhibition of malignant tumours in mice, even after they had spread widely. There has been recent difficulty in confirming all claims, but the subject remains a potentially exciting one. Several other fragments of normal body proteins, not themselves anti-angiogenic, have also been found to have anti-angiogenic activity (e.g. part of the hormone prolactin)[5].

Angiogenesis and anti-angiogenesis is normally a nicely balanced system in all tissues (Fig. 35). For a given blood oxygen content, blood vessels will continue to grow until the needs of a tissue or organ are fully met, after which the angiogenic stimulus is shut off and angiostatic factors turned on. There is currently a fast rate of discovery of new stimulating and inhibiting factors. The large numbers of names and abbreviations is very confusing to entrants to this field. But to an onlooker like myself it appears that cancer research may be in the process of changing its direction or, at least, its emphasis, in an extraordinarily interesting way.

Other requirements for the successful spread of tumours include increased extracellular matrix degradation by tumour- and host-secreted proteases (enzymes which can destroy protein), actual

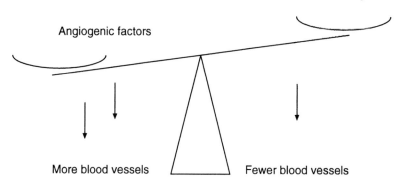

Figure 35 Cartoon emphasising that the density of blood vessels in any tissue is a balance between factors encouraging and factors inhibiting blood vessel growth.

movement or migration of cells into host tissues, and reduction of cell-to-cell adhesion. In addition, apoptosis (see p. 75) has to be switched off or inhibited before unrestrained cell growth becomes possible.

In years to come many of the mysteries of cancer will be solved, though others will doubtless appear. The sort of mystery which studies of angiogenesis may help to solve is exemplified by a patient of mine who had a 'radical mastectomy' to remove a cancer of the breast, leaving a long scar over the site of her breast. (This unpleasant and mutilating operation has now been mostly abandoned, because careful controlled trials have shown that equally good results can in most cases be achieved with much less radical surgery.) My patient remained well for five years, with no signs of recurrence of the tumour, until she had an attack of pneumonia, whereupon multiple individual nodules of cancerous tissue started growing all along the scar. In retrospect, it seems likely that a lot of individual cancer cells had been scattered in the wound during the initial operation, but that they had insufficient blood supply to multiply and grow. Then along came an infection which produced a lot of stimulatory circulating cytokines which switched on angiogenesis and got all the tiny lumps of residual tumour growing again.

Another patient, a man of 50, was sent to me with multiple circular shadows, about ¾ inch in diameter, visible all over the lung fields in a chest X-ray. Other evidence suggested that he had an underlying cancer of the bowel which had 'metastasised' (i.e. spread to distant sites) to the lungs. He felt well; so well, indeed, that he refused to give permission for one of the presumed tumour nodules to be removed

210

and examined under the microscope, though there could be no reasonable doubt that he had multiple lumps of a malignant tumour of some sort. I watched him at increasingly long intervals with chest X-rays for about ten years until I left my clinical service at St. Bartholomew's Hospital in London. The tumour nodules never got any bigger, but never went away. It seems in retrospect likely that some powerful angiostatic factor stopped the tumours spreading. Unhappily such phenomena are extremely rare. This is the only example I have ever seen myself of spontaneous arrest of already widely spread tumours. But however rare such occurrences may be, they give us hope that at least some cancers may eventually prove to be controllable by anti-angiogenic therapy. As I write, the first human trials of this type of therapy are getting under way.

Other aspects of angiogenesis

All I have done in this chapter is to introduce some of the many remaining mysteries about cancer. There is an interesting shift in research away from exclusive concentration on identifying the genetic make-up of malignant cells towards understanding how such cells can invade normal tissues and secure themselves a blood supply when they do. Such studies overlap with many aspects of physiology. For example, each month an egg (ovum) is shed from a fertile woman's ovary and is conveyed to the womb (see p. 103). New tissue starts growing in the bed of the egg in the ovary, forming the 'corpus luteum' (Latin: 'yellow body'). This shrivels up if the egg is not fertilised; but if it is the corpus luteum continues to grow. It provides hormones which support the first three months or so of the pregnancy. There is much current interest in the interplay of angiogenic and angiostatic factors in the growth and shrivelling up of each corpus luteum. VEGF and its receptors have been identified as playing a major role, as has insulin-like growth factor (IGF) and its receptors. Sex steroids play some part in angiogenesis of new lining tissue (endometrium) of the womb at the beginning of the menstrual cycle. They also shut down endometrial blood vessels if pregnancy does not occur, so that endometrium is shed. This latter action is made use of in hormone replacement therapy (HRT). For example, 17-αhydroxyprogesterone derivatives incorporated in HRT preparations prevent undue endometrial growth by shutting down uterine blood vessels.

New blood vessel formation is also an important factor in the healing of all but the smallest wounds. The excessive formation of new blood vessels in the retina of the eye in diabetes is nowadays the commonest cause of acquired blindness. I have already outlined in Chapter 7 my reasons for suggesting that PDGF may be the immediate cause of clubbing of the fingers, in which excessive growth of blood vessels in the finger pulp is a characteristic feature. As I mentioned in Chapter 8, angiogenesis is a necessary part of the formation of pannus in rheumatoid joints. There is current interest in the possibility of limiting joint damage by preventing pannus formation by angiostatic interventions. Angiogenesis is also relevant to the formation of atheroma, the cholesterol-rich deposits which narrow and obstruct large arteries and which are the main cause of heart attacks and strokes. Angiogenesis is necessary for new small blood vessels to grow in blood vessel walls and also to nourish the damaging lump of atheroma and allow it to grow. Drug or dietary treatment of arterial disease can directly lessen atheroma plaques and at the same time reduce the number of new blood vessels in the plaques.

Summary

The study of new blood vessel formation is a very fast-moving field at present. Angiogenesis is involved in many processes (e.g. in wound healing, in the growth and decay of the ovarian corpus luteum in women's reproductive life and in the formation of destructive pannus in rheumatoid joints). Recently there has been great interest in the possibilities of inhibition of growth of new blood vessels in cancer. Since no tumour can get to a damaging size unless it has an adequate blood supply, there is enormous current excitement about the possibilities of anti-angiogenic treatments. At present this approach looks (to me) as if it might even match or overtake drugs which directly attack and kill cancer cells.

Anti-angiogenic drugs may act directly, or perhaps by the subtle but so far rather disappointing 'anti-sense' approach[6] in which synthetic DNA fragments are designed to combine with and inactivate a damaging gene. Anti-angiogenesis treatment may also interfere with normal wound healing, and with the processes of recovery from blocked arteries in the heart and elsewhere.

An anti-cancer treatment designed to prevent tumours getting an adequate blood supply has to be very selective to interfere with the damaging formation of new blood vessels supplying tumours without interfering with important normal functions, but results in animals using this approach look promising. Watch this space!

22

MOTOR NEURONE DISEASE

People all over the world have been working on the problem of motor neurone disease (MND) for more than 50 years, but it remains unsolved. I shall review a lot of published work in this last chapter because I want to use MND as an example of the enormous number of interconnecting lines of evidence which sometimes have to be examined in attempts to understand a common condition. I have looked after many people with motor neurone disease but have never done any relevant personal research on the disease. The only possible advantage I might claim for this review is that it starts from no particular point of view, though inevitably I have developed an opinion of my own about the disease.

MND is a progressive and fatal disease of the spinal cord and/or the brain[1]. It affects both 'upper' and 'lower' motor neurones (defined in Chapter 3: see p. 21). Fig. 4 (see p. 22) shows the main routes of upper and lower motor neurones. The commonest form of MND is Amyotrophic Lateral Sclerosis (ALS)[*] in which both upper and lower motor neurones are involved. Less common varieties of MND are progressive (myelopathic) muscular atrophy, in which the lower motor neurones in the spinal cord are principally involved, and (progressive) bulbar palsy, in which the lower parts of the brain supplying the tongue and swallowing muscles are chiefly affected. Because ALS is much the commonest variety of MND the diagnosis nearly always means that the victim had ALS.

Many famous people have suffered from motor neurone disease – in recent years the late David Niven, James Mason and Jill Tweedie.

Some 5–10% of people with MND report that someone in the immediate family had or has the condition. In many, probably most, of these rare familial cases the disease is passed on as an autosomal

---

[*] This particular Greek mouthful is descriptive: 'a-' = without; '-myo-' = muscle; 'troph-' = nourishment (implying that the muscles become wasted); 'lateral sclerosis' = the side parts of the spinal cord which become hard or thickened from disease.

dominant[*]. But in the majority of cases the disease is sporadic, i.e. it arises in families without any affected relatives and appears to strike at random. Such sporadic non-genetic cases make up the great majority. But since familial cases behave clinically in a similar way to sporadic cases (in terms of speed of deterioration and in selectivity of affected neurones), study of familial cases might shed some light on the possible cause or causes.

Men are about 1½ times more commonly affected than women. Somewhere between 3 and 14 per 100,000 population are affected at any one time. MND has an incidence comparable with that of multiple sclerosis (see Chapter 3), but the number of sufferers alive at any one time is much less because the lifespan of MND is so short. All varieties of MND account for around 1 in 100,000 deaths per year in most populations. No notable racial differences have been identified but the disease is commoner in whites than in blacks. Skilled non-manual workers have the highest incidence, but differences between social classes are small. There are some geographical differences in incidence, though it is not certain whether the disease in Japan and in some Far East islands (Guam in particular) is the same as in other parts of the world.

The clinical course of MND

The disease causes weakness and eventually paralysis of the muscles supplied by the affected neurones. This most commonly starts in the leg muscles but later other muscles concerned with breathing and swallowing may be affected. The eye muscles are usually spared. Death usually results from paralysis of breathing, or from pneumonia. The disease runs an inexorable course. It lasts about 2½ years from first symptoms to death, though longer survivals are possible. Only about 15% of sufferers live as long as five years from first diagnosis. The disease seems to progress more rapidly in older than in younger people. Artificial support of breathing, eating and other bodily functions can extend life, though most sufferers choose not to accept such options even when they are available. Although intellectual function may become impaired, in many cases it remains normal throughout the illness, though careful studies reveal minor faults in intellectual functions and language in some patients[2]. Everyone knows

---

[*] 'Autosomal' refers to inheritance which is independent of the sex of the affected person; 'dominant' is defined elsewhere (see p. 60). The obverse of 'autosomal' is 'sex-linked'. As its name suggests it involves the sex chromosomes. Colour blindness and haemophilia are sex-linked, and only occur in males.

of the intellectual scientific achievements of Stephen Hawking, the theoretical physicist. Much of his recent work has been done despite his inability to speak, swallow, or move almost any muscle in his body. There is an allied disease in which the typical motor paralysis is associated with dementia from the onset of the illness, but this is less common than classic MND.

The disease can strike from the age of about 40 onwards; 62 is the commonest age at death. There may have been a slight increase in death rates from MND in the last few decades, but this may be due to better diagnosis and the increasing age of the population. Although some data suggest that the longer you live the greater your chance of getting the disease, other data suggest that 55–75 are the years of maximal risk and that the risk declines after 75[3].

Some studies have suggested that preceding severe mechanical trauma to the head or neck may be commoner in MND patients than in a control population of similar age. In animals, trauma can initiate damage to neurones which can be alleviated with nerve growth factors. In man, the evidence that trauma plays a significant part in MND remains controversial[4,5]. Previous vigorous physical activity has been said to be associated with MND[6].

Pathological changes in MND

The cell bodies of motor neurones bear the brunt of the disease. Conduction of impulses in the thin nerve fibres themselves usually remains normal until late in the disease, though a sub-group of ALS patients have conduction abnormalities in motor nerves. Under the microscope motor neurone cell bodies show several abnormalities[7]. Swellings looking like filaments or microtubules are common. These are 10–15nm in diameter, about one thousandth of the diameter of a single human red blood cell. The filamentous swellings are in loosely arranged bundles (skeins). They are sometimes seen in both motor nerve cell bodies and in nerve fibres[8]. They contain a specific protein, ubiquitin (Latin: 'ubique' = everywhere) whose function seems to be to latch onto other proteins, thereby marking them down for removal by the so-called ubiquitin-proteolytic pathway[9].

Other abnormal collections of material inside cells (cellular 'inclusions') are seen almost invariably in MND, but only rarely in other neurological disorders[10], apart from the neurofibrillary skeins and tangles in Alzheimer's disease (see Chapter 9), and Lewy bodies in Parkinson's disease[11]. In MND 'Bunina bodies' are usually visible in the lower motor neurone nuclei in the spinal cord and brain stem.

215

They can be appropriately dyed and identified under the microscope and are reliable markers of MND when present[12]. These strange microscopic objects do not look like either viruses or bacteria. Bunina bodies appear to be abnormal collections of proteinaceous material[13], some of which is ubiquitin[9]. This is known to bind strongly to the metal element aluminium – though concentrations of aluminium are not increased in nerve cells in ALS[14]. The presence of discrete Bunina bodies containing ubiquitin suggests that there is some intra-nuclear material which has been marked down for degradation by its combination with ubiquitin, but which cannot be processed normally. This therefore accumulates and damages nerve cells.

A better understood type of abnormal cell inclusion is found in nerve cell nuclei in Huntington's disease in man and in the genetically-engineered mouse which is bred to express abnormal (mutant) Huntington's genes. Apart from the presence of inclusion bodies in neurones, Huntington's disease resembles MND only in that it is a relentlessly progressive human brain disease of middle age. It is associated with dementia and bizarre muscle movements. It is a hereditary disease in which the genetic fault involves an excess of so-called 'triplet repeats' of (technically speaking) the CAG code in the DNA of a specific chromosome (the short arm of chromosome 4). This instructs the cell to make a protein which is abnormally lengthened by a string of glutamine residues. The protein cannot be metabolised normally. It therefore accumulates as intracellular particles which eventually cause nerve cell damage or destruction[15,16]. This can be due to aggregation of the particles themselves, or to promotion of aggregation with other proteins. Despite the combination with ubiquitin, it seems that cells cannot process the material. Several other conditions causing nerve or muscle disorders are also caused by the 'triplet-repeat' type of genetic fault but there is no evidence of a similar fault in sporadic MND.

Chemically[17] and under the electron microscope[18] Bunina bodies resemble the structure inside cells known as the 'rough endoplasmic reticulum'. (Although the word 'reticulum' means a net, the endoplasmic reticulum is really more like a collapsed balloon, with a cavity surrounded by a membrane. It is concerned with the folding and processing of newly synthesised proteins.) Other 'hyaline' (Greek: 'hyalos' = glass; i.e. glassy) ubiquitin-containing inclusions may also be present. These have been reported in both familial as well as sporadic MND[12]. All these cellular inclusions might suggest that neurones in MND have been suffering from excessive protein degradation; but the concentrations in spinal cord tissue of all known enzymes concerned with protein degradation appear to be normal[19]. It seems more sensible to regard the presence of intra-cellular inclusions as evidence that nerve cells are producing insoluble lumps of protein which cannot be degraded by cellular enzymes. It is also reasonable to assume that such inclusions interfere with nerve cell function.

Affected neurones seem to become apoptotic[20]. The body is somehow signalled to accept this form of cell death and not to provoke an inflammatory response to resist it. There is some evidence which suggests that apoptosis-promoting gene(s) may be overactive in MND[21], but nothing to suggest why they should be switched on. The cytokine known as TNFα is increased in the cerebrospinal fluid of MND patients. It may mediate or accelerate neuronal cell death by apoptosis in MND[22].

Cause

'A unifying hypothesis will have to explain the diverse geographical occurrence, clinical features, and selective vulnerability and relative resistance of different neuronal populations in the disease. ... Viruses, metals, endogenous toxins, immune dysfunction, endocrine abnormalities, impaired DNA repair, altered axonal transport, and trauma have all been etiologically linked with ALS, but convincing research evidence of a causative role for any of these factors is yet to be demonstrated'[23].

Many investigators have pointed to resemblances between three common neurological disorders which all occur at a similar time of life: MND, Alzheimer's disease (see Chapter 9) and Parkinson's disease. In some reported cases, two have occurred together[24]. The epidemiological resemblances have suggested that all three conditions might result from defective resistance of cell constituents to oxidative damage from 'free radicals'[25,26] – highly reactive chemicals produced during metabolism (see below). In Alzheimer's disease the protein ubiquitin accumulates inside cells (see p. 82) as it does in MND, but is contained in so-called 'neurofibrillary tangles' rather than in hyaline or skein-like inclusions.

The way in which previously normal individuals can be struck down by these diseases in their fifties or sixties has suggested the possibility that age-related attrition of neurones may be superimposed on some subtle damage arising early in life[27]. Such a theory may eventually prove to be true, but it is rather unhelpful since there is no obvious way in which it can at present be tested.

A specific enzyme defect

There is now much evidence that familial cases are linked to point mutations in the gene which codes in nerve cells for a specific enzyme, a protein catalyst called copper-zinc superoxide dismutase (Cu/Zn SOD). The enzyme concerned is one of a family which helps to inactivate and disable highly reactive and potentially damaging 'free radicals', chemicals produced during reactions involved in extracting energy from foodstuffs. Technically, free radicals are chemical species containing one or more unpaired electrons. This makes them highly reactive. The most damaging is the hydroxyl radical, but a number of other chemical species are also important. There is evidence of hydroxyl radical damage to brain neurones in many cases of dementia, though not in all the neurodegenerative diseases. One important school of thought, impressed by the clinical and pathological similarities between Parkinson's disease, Alzheimer's disease and MND, has suggested that in all three conditions nerve cells are damaged by the accumulation of superoxide radicals.

The gene for Cu/Zn SOD resides on chromosome 21 in the 21q22.1 band[28]. Each molecule of the enzyme concerned contains one zinc and one copper atom. These are intimately concerned with the enzyme's chemical function. Many different mutations have been recognised. Most result in a dominant type of inheritance of MND, but an autosomal recessive variety has also been recognised[29]. On the face of it, it is odd that many diverse differences in the protein structure of an enzyme can give rise to the same clinical manifestations. The reason seems to be that many minor alterations in protein shape can interfere with the metal binding sites in the molecule[30]. It is also odd that such a biochemical disease should often show itself in heterozygotes, i.e. in people whose cells contain only a single copy of the defective enzyme. In most situations of this sort half the normal amount of an enzyme will usually only produce mild if any symptoms. A recent extraordinary observation is that mice in which Cu/Zn SOD has been removed ('knocked out') by genetic manipulation appear to be entirely normal. It may therefore be that it is not the impaired removal of superoxide by defective Cu/Zn SOD which causes the damage in MND, but rather the acquisition of a toxic gain of function by the mutant protein (see below). The selective vulnerability of motor neurones in the presence of SOD mutations is a only a relative phenomenon – that is, it is not a 'black or white' affair. Careful examination has shown abnormalities in other parts of the nervous system (e.g. in pathways concerned with sensation rather than movement).

Human genes can be grafted into mice, creating so-called 'transgenic' animals. Human neurofilament genes inserted into mice make the animals develop neurological defects and abnormal filamentous swellings in nerve cells resembling those of human ALS[31]. Other transgenic mice have been created having the mutation in the gene coding for SOD-1 which causes human familial MND. These mice also develop neurological defects resembling ALS[32].

As mentioned above, an interesting recent suggestion has emerged from these studies: that mutations in the Cu/Zn SOD gene may have created an inverted, anomalous and toxic gain of function rather than a loss of function. Instead of mopping up damaging free radicals, the altered enzyme might actually produce free radicals[33]. Various hypotheses can explain how a gain of enzyme function might arise and how abnormal handling of free radicals by mutant SOD-1 might increase the formation of highly damaging peroxynitrite or hydroxyl free radicals. Cellular toxicity might result from release of copper or zinc, or from abnormal protein deposits resulting from aggregation of the defective SOD-1 protein. Concentrations of the SOD-1 enzyme have been measured in brain and in various other tissues in sporadic MND. They are not abnormal – though a related free radical scavenger enzyme (glutathione peroxidase) may be reduced in ALS[34].

Horses carry a gene closely similar to the human Cu/Zn SOD gene. They can also suffer from an inherited condition similar to ALS. Motor neurones in their spinal cord show abnormal structures in nerve cells which resemble Bunina bodies, though these are not the same as in man[35]. Unfortunately the SOD gene in these diseased horses appears to be identical with that in normal animals[36], so horse ALS is clearly not the same condition as human inherited MND.

MND runs in families in 5–10% of cases. Mutations in the SOD gene account for 20% of familial cases and about 2% of all cases of MND. But neither in the human sporadic cases of MND nor in inherited MND in horses is there commonly a recognisable defect in the enzyme, although a few specific mutations have been reported in apparently sporadic human cases[37]. A technique known as 'linkage analysis' has revealed that human chromosomes 2q and 9q may contain genes, mutations of which may underlie some rare forms of juvenile MND[1]. But no genetic predisposition has so far been identified in the great majority of human MND sufferers.

Other possible causes

Many investigators have speculated that MND might be caused by some mineral deficiency (e.g. of calcium, magnesium, copper or iodine – to name only a few elements). But mineral supplementation does not help. The largely negative findings 'suggest that generation of free radicals from exogenous chemicals is not important in ALS, and further that the neurone (as compared with other cell types) is poorly protected against the toxicity of hydrogen peroxide'[38]. It is striking that the MND seen in Guam and related Pacific islands is associated, like sporadic MND, with Bunina bodies and skein-like inclusions[39]. No one yet knows why these structures appear. If they are simply produced when motor nerve cells degenerate and can appear in various different varieties of MND they may not necessarily tell us anything at all about its underlying cause. On the other hand, Bunina bodies are virtually diagnostic of MND and are almost never seen in other neurodegenerative conditions.

Auto-immune dysfunction

Many diseases in man are known to be 'auto-immune' – that is, caused by the body reacting against its own cells in a damaging way. In some people dying from ALS an excess of lymphocytes has been seen in the spinal cord, suggesting immunological damage[40]. Degeneration of motor nerve cells can be produced by inoculating animals with spinal cord 'grey matter'. This contains the cell bodies of lower motor neurones and provokes an immune reaction ('auto-immune grey matter disease') which damages both upper and lower motor neurones, producing muscle weakness similar to that of MND in man[41]. The foci of damage in the recipient animals' spinal cords look similar to lesions of MND in man. However, the evidence for a comparable immune reaction in human MND is not strong. It is possible to show the presence of antibodies and increased chemical neurotransmitter release in mouse motor neurones after injecting the mice with serum from ALS patients, but not after injecting serum from normal people[42]. This also suggests that an immunological reaction could be damaging. But this is a long way from creating an animal model of MND. Most human auto-immune diseases respond in some degree to so-called 'immunosuppressive' drugs such as steroids and azathioprine, but such drugs have been given for a year to ALS patients with no discernible benefit[43].

Multifocal motor neuropathy with conduction block (MMNCB) is a rare condition with some features resembling MND, though MND can be distinguished by the absence, until late stages, of nerve conduction block. MMNCB is presumably immune-mediated, because the neurological features of motor weakness and paralysis often improve spectacularly with high doses of immunoglobulins[44]. Unfortunately MND is not improved by this treatment.

220

Virus infections

Since acute poliomyelitis (formerly called 'infantile paralysis') is known to be due to an infection with the polio virus, which particularly attacks lower motor neurone cells in the spinal cord, it is natural to speculate that some similar virus might selectively attack upper as well as lower motor neurones and cause MND. However, searches for polio virus infection in ALS have so far drawn a blank[45]. In any case, poliomyelitis has been gone from the developed world for almost a decade because of the great success of vaccination. MND incidence has not altered.

Inoculating monkeys with another virus (technically a 'togavirus') has produced neurological defects resembling ALS[46]. Some genetically susceptible wild mice develop a progressive MND, after a long latent period, when infected by a specific virus[47], but no comparable virus has been identified in human MND[48]. One objection to invoking a virus cause is the natural history of MND. This is a relentlessly progressive condition. Although an acute attack of poliomyelitis can be devastating, once the patient has recovered the pattern of muscular paralysis usually remains constant for the rest of life. None the less, other viruses are capable of producing a grumbling rather than an acute infection (e.g. hepatitis C). As I discussed in Chapter 3, multiple sclerosis may well be caused by a low-grade persisting virus infection acquired decades before the disease becomes manifest.

Deficiency of nerve growth or nerve protective factors

Another chase which seems to have petered out is the investigation of various nerve growth factors – chemical stimulants which cause neurones to grow and to sprout fibre connections. So far there is no evidence that the known nerve growth factors are deficient in MND.

Instead of incriminating some damaging neurotoxic factor, is MND due perhaps to the absence of some neuroprotective factor? During development of the brain and spinal cord some neurones are cleared away by apoptosis while others are stimulated to grow, by chemical 'neurotrophic' factors, of which at least four separate ones have already been identified[49]. This avenue is still being actively explored. There is current interest in gene products called 'Brn-3a' which appear to give nerve cells in culture some protection against apoptosis. Indirect protection of nerve cells is also given by angiostatic factors such as those discussed in the last chapter, because the survival and growth of nerve cells is only possible if cells retain an adequate blood supply. One of the growth factors mentioned above is a protein called 'ciliary neurotropic factor' (CNTF) which has been observed to improve the survival of several types of nerve cell cultured outside the body. It has been tried experimentally as a possible treatment for MND, but has too many adverse side-effects. Its distribution in the body of MND patients has thrown up the surprising finding that it is present in unusually high concentration in the skin, perhaps as a response to the disease process[50]. There is a very curious observation that patients with MND almost never get bedsores, even though they are grossly enfeebled towards the end of their lives and lie still for long periods. It has therefore been suggested that CNTF may in some way protect against bedsores.

Extrinsic toxic agents

Various metals have been suspected of being causal agents (e.g. lead, aluminium, selenium and many others). Some seem to be taken up selectively by motor neurones, making them plausible causes of MND, (e.g. inorganic mercury[51]). Unfortunately there is no evidence of excess of mercury or of any other element in the brain, apart from aluminium. Acid rain can liberate large amounts of aluminium in a bioavailable form[52]. So far all searches for environmental aluminium have been negative, though it is interesting that chronic inflammation of the spinal cord resembling MND can be produced in rabbits by long-term low dose administration of aluminium. Aluminium toxicity in man has been seen in some patients with kidney failure inadvertently given aluminium. It involves bone and blood disorders as well as the nervous system. Since MND is not directly associated with either bone or blood disorders, aluminium toxicity seems unlikely to be its cause.

Could the neuronal damage be due to a common external organic damaging agent? Two examples of neurotoxic materials causing human disease are lathyrism and cassavism. These two conditions are both examples of irreversible spastic paralysis caused by eating staple diets of grass pea and cassava root, respectively. Mildewed sugar cane can produce brain damage and muscle disorder. The cycad seed kernel, containing the neurotoxin cycasin, is thought to have a role in causing the variety of Parkinsonism/dementia-associated ALS which is found in the Western Pacific[53]. A clue to the possible involvement of such an agent is that spouses of affected patients appear to have an increased risk of ALS[53]. Deficiency of calcium and magnesium has been suggested as perhaps magnifying the neurotoxic effects of harmful dietary constituents.

One report has suggested an increased incidence of MND in farmers[54]. Considerable impetus has been given to the search for an ingested toxic factor in MND by the discovery that an agricultural chemical called MPTP can produce in man a picture virtually identical with the common neurodegenerative condition known as Parkinson's disease. In 1942 in Italy there was an epidemic of combined lower and upper motor neurone damage, without sensory loss, which closely resembled ALS. The condition was eventually traced to organophosphate poisoning from a rubbish dump close to a farmyard. But once the affected patients were isolated no further neurological damage ensued, though the disability persisted[55].

Poisoning by some specific article of diet does not adequately account for the progression of the disease. I have watched several sufferers from MND towards the end of their lives. They remain in hospitals or hospices, on standard diets. Despite this they continue to deteriorate relentlessly. I think therefore that MND is most unlikely to be due to a limited exposure to a toxin over a short time period. Organic compounds of mercury may be an exception. Bacteria can transform inorganic mercury into a fat-soluble organic form (methyl mercury)[56], which can induce neuronal apoptosis[57]. A single exposure to dimethyl mercury has been recorded as having caused long delayed brain damage in man. Perhaps we have yet to identify a poison which has the same progressively damaging effects as does dimethyl mercury. Cases of intolerance to specific foods (e.g. peanuts) are well-known, though not common. It therefore remains remotely possible that MND might be caused in a few specially susceptible individuals by a common article of diet such as potatoes. Continuing exposure to or ingestion of a common environmental or dietary factor could perhaps explain the relentless way in which MND behaves even in a protective hospital environment[58]. Although this seems to me most unlikely, it is exceedingly difficult to disprove.

The 'excitotoxic' theory

This currently popular theory implies that motor neurones are being damaged by being driven to discharge excessively[59]. Activation of neurones involves a series of complex chemical reactions leading to the entry of calcium ions into cells and to the release of calcium bound to an intracellular structure, the endoplasmic reticulum (see p. 216). The many observations of increased calcium concentrations in neurones and in motor nerve terminals in ALS are compatible with excessive activation[60]. Aberrant electrical excitation of heart muscle fibres in a circus manner is well known. It leads to failure of coordinated cardiac contraction and can even cause death by 'ventricular fibrillation'. One might therefore envisage the possibility that there is a comparable abnormal circular excitation going on in the brain in MND. If so, an increase in local metabolic rate and regional blood flow would be expected. But overall glucose consumption[61] and cerebral blood flow are both less than normal[62]. Regional blood flows in the frontal and anterior temporal regions and in the sensori-motor cortex are all reduced in MND[63,64]. On these grounds I do not believe that aberrant excessive circular excitation could possibly account for MND. Indeed, unless excessive neuronal activation could be identified in the early stages of MND, before neurones were supposedly 'exhausted', excito-toxic theories seem (to me) to be non-starters.

On the other hand, there is some evidence that MND patients do have excessive release of the ubiquitous excitant chemical neurotrans-mitter 'glutamate'. Excessive glutamate release might somehow have exhausted motor neurones. There is some evidence that glutamate transporters (chemicals which remove glutamate from the junctions between nerve cells, thus terminating its excitatory effect) are deficient in ALS. Reduced activity of these transporters seems the likeliest cause for a (compensatory) increased concentration of glutamate in the fluid surrounding the brain (the 'cerebrospinal') fluid. One of the active principles of the cycad seed (see below) is an amino acid which is a low potency activator of glutamate-requiring receptors. Observations of this kind have led to a trial of a drug (riluzole) which partly blocks gluta-mate release at nerve terminals, and decreases the rate at which motor nerve cells discharge electrical impulses. Riluzole has been thought to protect nerve cells from glutamate-induced damage. In one trial treated patients with ALS survived longer than untreated ones[65]. (The same drug is being tested for its possible benefit in Parkinson's disease.) There is also current interest in lithium, a chemical element which is extensively used to treat depression (especially manic-depression). This is also thought to work by interfering with glutamate action.

Does the cycad seed give us further clues about MND? Cycasin has been observed to interfere with glucose transport across cell walls, or into vesicles (minute fluid-filled bladders) inside cells[66]. Neurones are not supplied with nutrients directly from the bloodstream and do not make direct contact with blood vessels. Nutrients and oxygen get into nerve cells via the glial cells, which lie close to neurones. They can modify neuronal function (e.g. by altering the local concentration of calcium and of neurotransmitters such as glutamate). Very little is yet known about the function of glial cells in the brain, though (as I mentioned in Chapter 9) the neurofibrillary tangles which characterise damaged neurones in Alzheimer's disease are also seen in glial cells. Perhaps in MND glial cells become functionally inadequate in handling glucose or oxygen.

I recall that when I was a student no-one seemed to know what lymphocytes did, even though they comprised more than a third of all the white cells of the blood. Their vital role in immune protection was only discovered later. In the brain there are more glial cells than there are neurones. So glial cells must be immensely important, but we have very little idea what they do. I predict that one day they will be found to have some function which no one has yet envisaged. I hope I shall live long enough to see the revelation.

The brain in adult life is unique, amongst other organs, in relying exclusively on glucose for its energy supply. However, in fetal life, and in the newborn, the brain can use other sources of energy, particularly ketones – breakdown products of fat as well as of carbohydrates. In an indirect way I discovered that the brain also uses these alternative fuels in established and severe high blood pressure, as well as in cerebrovascular disease[67]. Since the adult brain can evidently adapt to use fuels other than glucose, might MND be helped by deliberately increasing the concentration of ketones in the blood? I have tried to find out whether diabetes, especially Type I, in which ketone excess is often present, gives any protection against MND; but the evidence is against this[68]. One old observation is interesting: reduced glucose metabolism was demonstrated in structurally normal brain cortex in MND, with normal neuronal numbers – suggesting that in MND some neurones 'exist in a state of neuronal nonfunction, rather than cell death'[69]. The suggestion has also been made that ALS might be due to an inadequate blood supply, for which there has been some evidence[70]; but this has yet to be confirmed. I find it difficult to believe that it can be a major factor. There are quite gross differences in the symptoms, signs and prognosis of MND and of cerebrovascular disease.

Recent work has shown that the rate of turnover of energy supplies in the human body is very rapid. Virtually all energy-requiring activities, such as muscle movement, glandular secretion or neuronal excitation, are fuelled by adenosine triphosphate (ATP). Its contained energy is released when it loses one of its three phosphate groups and becomes adenosine diphosphate (ADP). ATP can be regarded as a powerful rechargeable battery whose contained energy can be released at body temperature. Curiously the analogy is less far-fetched than it sounds. Energy is released by oxidative reactions in mitochondria, hundreds of which minute bodies are found in every cell of our bodies. Mitochondria extract energy by, in effect, burning up foodstuffs. Each mitochondrion uses the energy so produced to build up a negative electrical charge inside it of one tenth to one fifth of a volt. This charge can be regarded as a storehouse of energy. In the human adult at rest it can be estimated that ATP equivalent to half the body weight (35kg) is synthesised and broken down each day. Since the brain consumes about one fifth of the total energy breakdown of the body at rest, one may conclude that about 7kg (15 pounds weight) of ATP is synthesised by mitochondria in brain cells and broken down each day. Looked at this way it would seem that the brain's energy supplies must normally be extraordinarily robust. It is surprising that the energy supply fails so rarely.

Resemblance to the prion diseases

Some points of resemblance to the spongiform encephalopathies have been noted: the dual pattern of inherited and sporadic cases; the uniform prevalence of MND in different populations; the late onset of the disease (suggesting a long incubation period); neuronal loss without much inflammation; the link with copper through Cu/Zn SOD; the specific copper-binding sites in normal prion protein (which contains copper). But all attempts to produce neuronal damage in animals by inoculating fresh MND post-mortem material have failed. No lesions were seen in mice during 600 days of observation after inoculating them with human diseased neuronal material[71].

It still remains possible that a conformational change in the protein structure of Cu/Zn SOD has interfered with its function, specifically in the way in which body constituents bind to the zinc which forms part of the protein[30]. Such a possibility might seem ridiculous, except that the example of the prion diseases comes again to mind. In these diseases, such as scrapie in sheep, bovine spongiform encephalopathy in cows (BSE) and kuru in man, it appears that a normal body 'prion' protein product (PrPc) is somehow changed in molecular spatial structure – though not in its chemical constituents – and folds into one of 4 abnormal protein shapes (PrPsc) which prevents it being removed by proteinases (protein degrading enzymes). The abnormal protein then accumulates in nerve cells (perhaps by a process resembling crystallisation) and damages them[72]. Could Bunina bodies and intra-cellular skeins, containing ubiquitin and some other important molecules, also contain structurally altered protein without necessarily accumulating in large quantities as, for example, the starchy protein amyloid does in Alzheimer's disease? I have found no reports conclusively demonstrating that Bunina bodies contain either copper or zinc. Whether they do or not, there could be a conformational change in the non-metallic part of one of the SOD enzymes. A recent publication[73] has identified a mutation of Cu/Zn SOD-1 in mice which heads to rapid neurological deterioration. Tests with appropriate antibodies suggested that the glial cells of these mice contain both SOD-1 and ubiquitin, and that motor neurone cells contain SOD-1.

Proteins can have exceedingly complex three-dimensional structures. Sometimes (as in the case of prion proteins already mentioned) an abnormal protein may have the same chemical amino acid constituents as a normal protein but be folded in such a way that it behaves abnormally. It is now recognised that some so-called 'heat shock proteins' – proteins whose synthesis is enhanced by stresses such as a rise in temperature – act as 'chaperones'. This delightful word describes their function of controlling the appropriate folding of protein chains, during or immediately after their synthesis, thus preventing their sticky surfaces becoming glued together or aggregating[74,75]. Chaperones are usually found in the endoplasmic reticulum (see p. 216) inside cells[76]. One possible functional defect in MND therefore might be that in sporadic MND (the common form) a normal chaperone protein is deficient, or perhaps changed so that its normal assembling function is deranged. This might then account for the abnormal collection within neurones of proteinaceous material, forming Bunina bodies (specific for MND). Defects in genes coding for neurofilaments have been found to be associated with MND[77]. It seems possible that consequential aggregates of neurofilament proteins could be a main causal factor in such cases.

One notable observation has been made of affected neuronal populations in Alzheimer's disease and ALS. The affected neuronal populations are anatomically interconnected[78], suggesting that a damaging agent such as a virus or an abnormal protein might pass from affected cells to unaffected ones.

To my mind the most compelling reason for thinking that MND is a protein-conformational disorder is that although in familial MND cases (with positively identified mutations in the Cu/Zn SOD-1 gene) the supposedly 'defective' enzyme has normal biochemical activity in cell culture and in transgenic mouse studies but can still apparently cause neuronal damage characteristic of human MND[79]. When we also take into account that even a single copy of the defective Cu/Zn SOD-1 gene can result in a dominant form of inheritance, normal expectations of genetic biochemical disorders are confounded. Doctors have long been familiar with the situation where a homozygous disorder* causes disease, whereas an individual heterozygous for the condition is a 'carrier' who may suffer a little from minor aspects of the full-blown

---

* homozygous: carrying two copies of a specific gene; heterozygous: carrying only a single copy.

disease or may be entirely normal. Sickle-cell disease and fibrocystic disease are examples. By contrast, an unfortunate individual carrying only a single copy of the abnormal but still functional Cu/Zn SOD-1 gene may suffer and die from clinically typical MND.

Some unanswered questions

Do motor neurones use more energy that other neuronal types? If so, a general defect in neuronal function might pick them out.

Is there mitochondrial exhaustion in MND? Mitochondrial DNA is particularly susceptible to oxidative stress. Mitochondrial metabolism is a major source of potentially damaging free radicals. In addition, there is a normal age-dependent damage to and deterioration of respiratory enzymes[80,81].

Do the Japanese get less MND because they have a higher frequency of the mitochondrial Mt5178A gene[82], which seems to predispose to longevity? Is there an inverse relationship between Mt5178A and MND?

Can the high prevalence of MND in the Western Pacific, especially in the island of Guam, be explained by some local factor, such as the supply of trace elements, deficiency of calcium or magnesium, or an excess of some toxic metal (e.g. lead or mercury)?

Could there be associated secondary hyperparathyroidism[83]?

Are the abnormalities reported in glutamate[84] and glycine transport in MND relevant[85]?

Has electroconvulsive therapy been tried in MND, with the idea of interrupting damaging neural circuits? If so, was there any benefit?

Is there any evidence that before glucose consumption and electrical activity start to fall (as they are known to do in MND) there is a period of time in which both are increased – as might be expected by the 'excitotoxic theory'?

Deletions of the neuronal apoptosis inhibitory gene NAIP or another related gene is associated with proximal spinal muscular atrophy in childhood but so far no similar mutations have been found in MND. What other genes might control neural apoptosis?

Ubiquitin-positive skein-like inclusions, which may be precursors of Bunina bodies and Lewy-body inclusions, are seen in ALS neurones. This suggests that nerve cells may be in an early stage of neuronal degeneration. But if so, why does MND seem to be 'all or none'? We don't see 'mild' cases at all (I think): this makes exhaustion of enzyme chains less likely.

There is a striking contrast between MND and organophosphate poisoning. A conformational change in a protein might explain the inexorable progression of MND, as already suggested. In organophosphate poisoning the neurological signs and symptoms stop once the toxin had been removed. Is it fair to take the persistence and progressively damaging course of MND as evidence pointing more towards a virus cause or a prion?

Why do almost all the genetic mitochondrial disorders cause neural problems? Is this because of the immense energy requirements of the brain?

Is there more ubiquitin in MND cell bodies than in others? If not why not?

Do Bunina bodies contain Cu/Zn SOD? Is this why they are virtually specific for ALS? Could a prion-like process lead to loss of function of this dismutase inside cells? If the dismutase is in Bunina bodies, then perhaps, despite nerve cells having otherwise normal cell constituents, might the enzyme be non-functional?

Is the recently identified NF-H mouse gene (also identified in MND) damaging, by making neurones produce too many filaments?

The Brn-3A transcription factor is a powerful stimulant of nerve filament growth[86]. Is this overexpressed in MND? If not, why not?

What do glial cells do? Why are there so many of them? Why cannot neurones get their energy supplies directly from nearby blood vessels without the intervention of glial cells?

Summary

Motor neurone disease (MND), the commonest variety of which is amyotrophic lateral sclerosis, is a disease of the middle-aged and elderly. It particularly impairs muscle function by damaging the spinal cord and brain stem, but it usually spares sensation and may leave intellect unimpaired. Over a course of about 30 months there is progressive paralysis of skeletal muscles leading in the end to failure of the respiratory muscles and death. The lower motor neurones in the spinal cord are commonly affected first, but later upper motor neurone bodies may also be involved. Nerve cell bodies contain typical inclusions known as Bunina bodies which are almost specific for MND.

Between 5% and 10% of all cases are hereditary. Some 20% of these cases can be firmly linked with many different inherited defects in an intracellular enzyme known as copper/zinc superoxide dismutase-1 (Cu/Zn SOD-1). This is thought to prevent damage from superoxide radicals, which are generated in mitochondria during the extraction of energy from foodstuffs. The remaining 90–95% of cases

229

of MND are sporadic and the concentration and chemical properties of the dismutase enzyme are normal.

Some features of MND suggest the possibility that it could be a disease involving a conformational change in some nerve cell protein, even in part of the Cu/Zn SOD-1 enzyme itself which perhaps becomes abnormally folded and unduly stable. Though not destroying its enzymic function such a protein might become less soluble and immune from identification and removal by the ubiquitin-proteolytic pathway. Such a change might then induce similar conformational changes in the enzyme in adjacent cells, with consequent functional damage. This is only one theory among many. At the present time there is no agreement between competing theories. Though we already know a lot about what is going on in MND, cure or even control of it still seem a long way off.

REFERENCES

CHAPTER 1

1. O'Malley JW (editor). In Praise of Medicine. In: Erasmus: Collected Works. 1989; Toronto: Toronto University Press.

CHAPTER 2

1. Platts-Mills TA, Tovey ER, Mitchell EB, et al. Reduction of bronchial hyperreactivity during prolonged allergen avoidance. Lancet 1982; 2: 675–678.
2. Schreck R, Albermann K, Baeuerle PA. Nuclear factor kappa B: an oxidative stress-responsive transcription factor of eukaryotic cells. Free Radic Res Commun 1992; 17: 221–237.
3. Terada N, Maesako K, Hiruma K, et al. Diesel exhaust particulates enhance eosinophil adhesion to nasal epithelial cells and cause degranulation. Int Arch Allergy Immunol 1997; 114: 167–174.
4. Barnes PJ. Pathophysiology of asthma. Brit J Clin Pharmacol 1996; 42: 3–10.
5. Lipworth BJ. Leukotriene-receptor antagonists. Lancet 1999; 353: 57–62.
6. ISAAC. Worldwide variation in prevalence of symptoms of asthma, allergic rhinoconjunctivitis, and atopic eczema: ISAAC. Lancet 1998; 351: 1225–1232.
7. Yemaneberhan H, Bekele Z, Venn A, et al. Prevalence of wheeze and asthma and relation to atopy in urban and rural Ethiopia. Lancet 1997; 350: 85–90.
8. Lee HS, Yap J, Wang YT, et al. Occupational asthma due to unheated polyvinylchloride resin dust. Br J Ind Med 1989; 46: 820–822.
9. Moisan TC. Prolonged asthma after smoke inhalation: a report of three cases and a review of previous reports. Med 1991; 33: 458–461.
10. Nielsen J, Fahraeus C, Bensryd I, et al. Small airways function in workers processing polyvinyl chloride. Int Arch Occup Environ Health 1989; 61: 427–430.
11. Falk H, Portnoy B. Respiratory tract illness in meat wrappers. J Amer med Ass 1976; 235: 915–917.
12. Kogevinas M, Antö JM, Sunyer J, et al. European Community Respiratory Health Survey Study Group. Occupational asthma in Europe and

other industrialised areas: a population-based study. Lancet 1999; 353: 1750–1754.

CHAPTER 3

1. Gale CR, Martyn CN. Migrant studies in multiple sclerosis. Prog Neurobiol 1995; 47: 425–448.
2. McHatters GR, Scham RG. Bird viruses in multiple sclerosis: combination of viruses or Marek's alone?. Neurosci Lett 1995; 188: 75–76.
3. Perron H, Garson JA, Bedin F, et al. Molecular identification of a novel retrovirus repeatedly isolated from patients with multiple sclerosis. The Collaborative Research Group on Multiple Sclerosis. Proc Natl Acad Sci USA 1997; 94: 7583–7588.
4. Williams KC, Ulvestad E, Hickey WF. Immunology of multiple sclerosis. Clin Neurosci 1994; 2: 229–245.
5. Bansil S, Cook SD, Rohowsky-Kochan C. Multiple sclerosis: immune mechanism and update on current therapies. Ann Neurol 1995; 37(Suppl 1): S87–S101.
6. Trapp BD, Peterson J, Ransohoff RM, et al. Axonal transection in the lesions of multiple sclerosis. New Engl J Med 1998; 338: 278–285.

CHAPTER 4

1. Hainsworth R. Physiology and pathophysiology of syncope. In: Syncope in the older patient. 1996; London: Chapman & Hall.
2. Henry JP. On the Triggering Mechanism of Vasovagal Syncope. Psychosom Med 1984; 46: 91–93.
3. Öberg B, Thorén P. Increased Activity in Left Ventricular Receptors during Hemorrhage or Occlusion of Caval Veins in the Cat. A Possible Cause of the Vasovagal Reaction. Acta physiol scand 1972; 85: 164–172.
4. Hainsworth R. Reflexes From the Heart. Physiol Rev 1991; 71: 617–658.
5. Scherrer U, Vissing S, Morgan BJ, et al. Vasovagal syncope after infusion of a vasodilator in a heart-transplant patient. New Engl J Med 1990; 322: 602–604.
6. Dickinson CJ. Fainting precipitated by collapse-firing of venous baroreceptors. Lancet 1993; 342: 970–972.
7. Pearce JW, Henry JP. Changes in cardiac afferent nerve-fiber discharges induced by hemorrhage and adrenaline. Amer J Physiol 1955; 183: 650 (abstract).

CHAPTER 5

1. Aragane Y, Yamada H, Schwarz A, et al. Transforming growth factor-alpha induces interleukin-6 in the human keratinocyte cell line HaCaT mainly by transcriptional activation. J Invest Dermatol 1996; 106: 1192–1197.
2. Trembath RC, Clough RL, Rosbotham JL, et al. Identification of a major susceptibility locus on chromosome 6p and evidence for further disease loci revealed by a two stage genome-wide search in psoriasis. Hum Mol Genet 1997; 6: 813–820.
3. Henseler T. The genetics of psoriasis. J Am Acad Dermatol 1997; 37: S1–S11.
4. Wrone-Smith T, Nickoloff BJ. Dermal injection of immunocytes induces psoriasis. J Clin Invest 1996; 98: 1878–1887.
5. Ezepchuk YV, Leung DY, Middleton MH, et al. Staphylococcal toxins and protein A differentially induce cytotoxicity and release of tumor necrosis factor-alpha from human keratinocytes. J Invest Dermatol 1996; 107: 603–609.
6. Sayama K, Midorikawa K, Hanakawa Y, et al. Superantigen production by *Staphylococcus aureus* in psoriasis. Dermatology 1998; 196: 194–198.

CHAPTER 6

1. Fida R, Lyster DJ, Bywater RA, Taylor GS. Colonic migrating motor complexes (CMMCs) in the isolated mouse colon. Neugastroenterol Motil 1997; 9: 99–107.
2. Bell IR, Schwartz GE, Peterson JM, Amend D. Symptom and personality profiles of young adults from a college student population with self-reported illness from foods and chemicals. J Am Coll Nutr 1993; 12: 693–702.
3. Kingham JG, Dawson AM. Origin of chronic right upper quadrant pain. Gut 1985; 26: 783–788.
4. Orr WC, Crowell MD, Lin B, et al. Sleep and gastric function in irritable bowel syndrome: derailing the brain-gut axis. Gut 1997; 41: 390–393.
5. Sanger GJ. 5-Hydroxytryptamine and functional bowel disorders. Neuro-gastroenterol Motil 1996; 8: 319–331.
6. Bindslev-Jensen C. Food allergy. Brit med J 1998; 316: 1299–1302.
7. Lindberg G, Glia A, Nyberg B, Veress B. Lymphocytic ganglionitis – a new entity causing severe motility disorders of the gut. Gastroenterology 1999; 116: G4476 (short communication).

CHAPTER 7

1. Stoller JK, Moodie D, Schiavone WA, et al. Reduction of Intrapulmonary Shunt and Resolution of Digital Clubbing Associated with Primary Biliary Cirrhosis after Liver Transplantation. Hepatology 1990; 11: 54–58.
2. Dickinson CJ. The aetiology of clubbing and hypertrophic osteoarthropathy. Europ J clin Invest 1993; 23: 330–338.
3. Dickinson CJ, Martin JF. Megakaryocytes and platelet clumps as the cause of finger clubbing. Lancet 1987; ii: 1434–1435.
4. Fox SB, Day CA, Gatter KC. Association between platelet microthrombi and finger clubbing. Lancet 1991; 338(ii): 313–314 (letter).
5. Wood WG. Developmental haemopoiesis. In: Blood and its disorders (eds Hardisty RM, Weatherall DJ). 1982; Oxford: Blackwell.

CHAPTER 8

1. Moore TL, Dorner RW. Rheumatoid factors. Clin Biochem 1993; 26: 75–84.
2. Kirschfink M. Controlling the complement system in inflammation. Immunopharmacology 1997; 38: 51–62.
3. Gaston JSH. Role of T-cells in the development of arthritis. Clin Sci 1998; 95: 19–31.
4. Rosen A, Casciola-Rosen L, Ahern J. Novel packages of viral and self-antigens are generated during apoptosis. J exp Med 1995; 181: 1557–1561.
5. Depraetere V, Golstein P. Dismantling in cell death: molecular mechanisms and relationship to caspase activation. Scand J Immunol 1998; 47: 523–531.
6. Casciola-Rosen L, Rosen A. Ultraviolet light-induced keratinocyte apoptosis: a potential mechanism for the induction of skin lesions and autoantibody production in LE. Lupus 1997; 6: 175–180.
7. Krause A, Kamradt T, Burmester GR. Potential infectious agents in the induction of of arthritides. Curr Opin Rheumatol 1996; 8: 203–209.
8. Altschuler EL. *Parvovirus B19* and the pathogenesis of rheumatoid arthritis: a case for historical reasoning. Lancet 1999; 354: 1026–1027.
9. Silman A, Bankhead C, Rowlingson B, et al. Do new cases of rheumatoid arthritis cluster in time or in space? Int J Epidemiol 1997; 26: 628–634.

CHAPTER 9

1. Salehi A, Ravid R, Gonatas NK, Swaab DF. Decreased activity of hippo-campal neurons in Alzheimer's disease is not related to the presence of neurofibrillary tangles. J Neuropathol Exp Neurol 1995; 54: 704–709.
2. Carr DB, Goate A, Phil D, Morris JC. Current concepts in the pathogen-esis of Alzheimer's disease. Am J Med 1997; 103: 3S–10S.
3. Hsiao K, Chapman P, Nilsen S, et al. Correlative memory deficits, Aβ elevation, and amyloid plaques in transgenic mice. Science 1996; 274: 99–102.
4. Forloni G, Tagliavini F, Bugiani O, Salmona M. Amyloid in Alzheimer's disease and prion-related encephalopathies: studies with synthetic peptides. Prog Neurobiol 1996; 49: 287–315.
5. Schmidt ML, Lee VM, Forman M, et al. Monoclonal antibodies to a 100-kd protein reveal abundant Aβ-negative plaques throughout grey matter of Alzheimer's disease brains. Am J Pathol 1997; 151: 69–80.
6. Thome J, Kornhuber J, Munch G, et al. New hypothesis on etiopathogen-esis of Alzheimer syndrome. Advanced glycation end products (AGEs). [German]. Nervenarzt 1996; 67: 924–929.
7. Armstrong RA, Winsper SJ, Blair JA. Aluminium and Alzheimer's disease: review of possible pathogenic mechanisms. Dementia 1996; 7: 1–9.
8. Snowdon DA, Kemper SJ, Mortimer JA, et al. Linguistic ability in early life and cognitive function and Alzheimer's disease in late life. Findings from the Nun Study. J Amer med Ass 1996; 275: 528–532.
9. Stern Y, Gurland B, Tatemichi TK, et al. Influence of education and occupation on the incidence of Alzheimer's disease. J Amer med Ass 1994; 271: 1004–1010.
10. Whalley LJ, Thomas BM, McGonigal G, et al. Epidemiology of presenile Alzheimer's disease in Scotland (1974–88) I. non-random geographical variation. Br J Psychiatry 1995; 167: 728–731.
11. Edland SD, Silverman JM, Peskind ER, et al. Increased risk of dementia in mothers of Alzheimer's disease cases: evidence for maternal inheritance. Neurology 1996; 47: 254–256.

CHAPTER 10

1. Kanis JA. Pathophysiology and treatment of Paget's disease of bone. 1998; London: Dunitz.
2. Ebersole JL, Taubman MA, Smith DJ, et al. Human immune responses to oral microorganisms. II. Serum antibody responses to antigens from *Actinobacillus actinomycetemcomitans* and the correlation with localized juvenile periodontitis. J Clin Immunol 1983; 3: 321–331.
3. Zafiropoulos GG, Flores-de-Jacoby L, Hungerer KD, et al. Humoral

antibody responses in periodontal disease. J Periodontol 1992; 63: 80–86.

4. Dickinson CJ. The possible role of osteoclastogenic oral bacteria products in etiology of Paget's disease. Bone 2000; 26: 101–102.

5. Blix IJ, Hars R, Preus HR, Helgeland K. Entrance of *Actinobacillus actinomycetemcomitans* into HEp-2 cells in vitro. J Periodontol 1992; 63: 723–728.

6. Renier J-C, Audran M. Progression in length and width of Pagetic lesions, and estimation of age at disease onset. Rev Rhum (Engl Ed) 1997; 64: 35–43.

7. Wheeler TT, Alberts MA, Dolan TA, McGorray SP. Dental, visual, auditory and olfactory complications in Paget's disease of bone. J Am Geriatr Soc 1995; 43: 1384–1391.

8. Barry HC. Paget's disease of bone. 1969; Edinburgh: Livingstone.

CHAPTER 11

1. Kasule J, Chimbira THK. Endometriosis in African Women. Cent Afric J Med 1987; 33: 157–159.

2. Thomas EJ. Endometriosis, 1995 – confusion or sense?. Int J Gynaecol Obstet 1995; 48: 149–155.

3. Koninckx PR, Ide P, Vandenbroucke W, Brosens IA. New aspects of the pathophysiology of endometriosis and associated infertility. J Reprod Med 1980; 24: 257–260.

4. Darrow SL, Vena JE, Batt RE, et al. Menstrual cycle characteristics and the risk of endometriosis. Epidemiology 1993; 4: 135–142.

5. D'Hooghe TM. Clinical relevance of the baboon as a model for the study of endometriosis. Fertil Steril 1997; 68: 613–625.

6. Dickinson CJ. Could tight garments cause endometriosis? Brit J Obst Gynaec 1999; 106: 1003–1005.

7. Ulmsten U, Andersson KE. Multichannel intrauterine pressure recording by means of microtransducers. Acta Obstet Gynecol Scand 1979; 58: 115–120.

CHAPTER 12

1. Ayres JG, Flint N, Smith EG, et al. Post-infection fatigue syndrome following Q fever. Quart J Med 1998; 91: 105–123.

2. White PD, Grover SA, Kangro HO, et al. The validity and reliability of the fatigue syndrome that follows glandular fever. Psychol Med 1995; 25: 917–924.

3. Pearn JH. Chronic fatigue syndrome: chronic ciguatera poisoning. Med J Aust 1997; 166: 309–310.

4. Abbey SE, Garfinkel PE. Neurasthenia and chronic fatigue syndrome: the role of culture in the making of a diagnosis. Amer J Psychiat 1991; 148: 1638–1646.

5. Ichise M, Salit IE, Abbey SE, et al. Assessment of regional cerebral perfusion by 99Tcm-HMPAO SPECT in chronic fatigue syndrome. Nuclear Medicine Communications 1992; 13: 767–772.
6. Costa DC, Tannock C, Brostoff J. Brainstem perfusion is impaired in chronic fatigue syndrome. Quart J Med 1995; 88: 767–773.
7. Schwartz RB, Garada BM, Komaroff AL, et al. Detection of intracranial abnormalities in patients with chronic fatigue syndrome: comparison of MR imaging and SPECT. AJR: Am J Roentgen 1994; 162: 935–941.
8. Cope H, Pernet A, Kendall B, David A. Cognitive functioning and magnetic resonance imaging in chronic fatigue. Br J Psychiatry 1995; 167: 86–94.
9. Hess CW, Bassetti C. Neurology of consciousness and of consciousness disorders [German]. Schweiz Rundschau Med Praxis 1994; 83: 212–219.
10. Tirelli U, Chierichetti F, Tavio M, et al. Brain positron emission tomography (PET) in chronic fatigue syndrome: preliminary data. Am J Med 1998: 105: 54S–58S.
11. Bruno RL, Frick NM, Cohen J. Polioencephalitis, stress, and the etiology of post-polio sequelae. Orthopedics 1991; 14: 1269–1276.
12. Dickinson CJ. Chronic fatigue syndrome – aetiological aspects. Europ J clin Invest 1997; 27: 257–267.

CHAPTER 13

1. Sartor RB. Current concepts of the etiology and pathogenesis of ulcerative colitis and Crohn's disease. Gastroenterol Clin North Am 1995; 24: 475–507.
2. Anonymous. A case-control study of ulcerative colitis in relation to dietary and other factors in Japan. The Epidemiology Group of the Research Committee of Inflammatory Bowel Disease in Japan. J Gastroenterol 1995; 30(Suppl 8): 9–12.

CHAPTER 14

1. Ferrari MD. Migraine. Lancet 1998; 351: 1043–1051.
2. Shimomura T, Kowa H, Nakano T, et al. Platelet superoxide dismutase in migraine and tension-type headache. Cephalalgia 1994; 14: 215–218.
3. Ophoff RA, Terwindt GM, Vergouwe MN, et al. Familial hemiplegic migraine and episodic ataxia type-2 are caused by mutations in the Ca2+ channel gene CACNL1A4. Cell 1996; 87: 543–552.
4. Schmidt C. Migraine and cerebral blood flow during centrifugation. Lancet 1997; 350: 1145 (letter).

CHAPTER 15

1. Dickinson CJ. Neurogenic Hypertension 1965; Oxford: Blackwell Scientific Publications.

2. Dickinson CJ. Neurogenic Hypertension 1991; London: Chapman & Hall.
3. Mann A. Hypertension: psychological aspects and diagnostic impact in a clinical trial. Psychol Med 1984; Monograph Suppl.5.
4. Law CM, De Swiet M, Osmond C, et al. Initiation of hypertension *in utero* and its amplification throughout life. Brit med J 1993; 306: 24–27.
5. Medical Research Council Working Party. Course of blood pressure in mild hypertensives after withdrawal of long term antihypertensive treatment. Brit med J 1986; 293: 988–992.
6. Swales JD (editor). Textbook of Hypertension 1994; Oxford: Blackwell Scientific publications.

CHAPTER 16

1. Thompson JMA, Dickinson CJ. The relation between the excretion of sodium and water and the perfusion pressure in the isolated, blood-perfused, rabbit kidney, with special reference to the changes occurring in clip-hypertension. Clin Sci Mol Med 1976; 50: 223–236.
2. Guyton AC, Coleman TG, Granger HJ. Circulation: Overall regulation. Ann Rev Physiol 1972; 34: 13–46.
3. Dickinson CJ, Lawrence JR. A slowly developing pressor response to small concentrations of angiotensin: its bearing on the pathogenesis of chronic renal hypertension. Lancet 1963; i: 1354–1356.
4. Dickinson CJ, Yu R. Mechanisms Involved in the Progressive Pressor Response to Very Small Amounts of Angiotensin in Conscious Rabbits. Circulat Res 1967; 20/21(Suppl.II): II-157–II-163.
5. Yu R, Dickinson CJ. Neurogenic effects of angiotensin. Lancet 1965; ii: 1276–1277.
6. Muirhead EE. Renal vasodepressor mechanisms: the medullipin system. J Hypertension 1993; 11(Suppl.5): S53–S58.

CHAPTER 17

1. Haller H, Hempel A, Homuth V, et al. Endothelial-cell permeability and protein kinase C in pre-eclampsia. Lancet 1998; 351: 945–949.
2. Schobel HP, Fischer T, Heuszer K, et al. Preeclampsia – a state of sympathetic overactivity. N Engl J Med 1996; 335: 1480–1485.
3. Smarason AK, Sargent IL, Redman CW. Endothelial cell proliferation is suppressed by plasma but not serum from women with preeclampsia. Am J Obstet Gynecol 1996; 174: 787–793.
4. Brown MA. The physiology of pre-eclampsia. Clin Exp Pharmacol Physiol 1995; 22: 781–791.
5. Taylor RN. Review: immunobiology of preeclampsia. Am J Reprod Immunol 1997; 37: 79–86.
6. Robillard PY, Hulsey TC, Perianin J, et al. Association of pregnancy-

induced hypertension with duration of sexual cohabitation before conception. Lancet 1994; 344: 973–975.
7. Robillard PY, Hulsey TC, Alexander GR, et al. Paternity patterns and risk of preeclampsia in the last pregnancy in multiparae. J Reprod Immunol 1993; 24: 1–12.
8. Lie RT, Rasmussen S, Brunborg H, et al. Fetal and maternal contributions to risk of pre-eclampsia: population based study. Brit med J 1998; 316: 1343–1347.

CHAPTER 18

1. Giaid A, Yanagisawa M, Langleben D, et al. Expression of endothelin-1 in the lungs of patients with pulmonary hypertension. New Engl J Med 1993; 328: 1732–1739.
2. Morse JH, Jones AC, Barst RJ, et al. Mapping of familial primary pulmonary hypertension locus (PPH1) to chromosome 2q31-q32. Circulation 1997; 95: 2603–2606.

CHAPTER 19

1. Ralston DR, Marsh CB, Lowe MP, Wewers MD. Antineutrophil cytoplasmic antibodies induce monocyte IL-8 release. Role of surface proteinase-3, alpha1-antitrypsin, and Fcgamma receptors. J Clin Invest 1997; 100: 1416–1424.

CHAPTER 20

1. Botez MI, Cadotte M, Beaulieu R, et al. Neurologic disorders responsive to folic acid therapy. Canad med Ass J 1976; 115: 217–223.
2. Kamei T, Kohno T, Ohwada H, et al. Experimental study of the therapeutic effects of folate, vitamin A, and vitamin B12 on squamous metaplasia of the bronchial epithelium. Cancer 1993; 71: 2477–2483.
3. MRC Vitamin Study Research Group. Prevention of neural tube defects: results of the Medical Research Council Vitamin Study. Lancet 1991; 338: 131–137.
4. Yates JR, Ferguson-Smith MA, Guzman-Rodriquez R, et al. Is disordered folate metabolism the basis for the genetic predisposition to neural tube defects? Clin Genet 1987; 31: 279–287.
5. Dickinson CJ. Does folic acid harm people with vitamin B12 deficiency? Quart J Med 1995; 88: 357–364.
6. Wild J, Schorah CJ, Sheldon TA, Smithells RW. Investigation of factors influencing folate status in women who have had a neural tube defect-affected infant. Brit J Obst Gynaec 1993; 100: 546–549.

7. Oakley GP. Folic Acid – Preventable Spina Bifida and Anencephaly. J Amer med Ass 1993; 269: 1292–1293.

CHAPTER 21

1. Dickinson CJ. Cardiovascular system. In: The Encyclopaedia of Medical Ignorance (eds Duncan R, Weston-Smith M) 1984; pp. 107–115. Oxford: Pergamon Press.
2. Wong AL, Haroon ZA, Werner S, et al. Tie2 expression and phosphorylation in angiogenic and quiescent adult tissues. Circ Res 1997; 81: 567–574.
3. Olson TA, Mohanraj D, Roy S, Ramakrishnan S. Targeting the tumor vasculature: inhibition of tumor growth by a vascular endothelial growth factor-toxin conjugate. Int J Cancer 1997; 73: 865–870.
4. O'Reilly MS, Holmgren L, Shing Y, et al. Angiostatin: A novel angiogenesis inhibitor that mediates the suppression of metastases by a Lewis lung carcinoma. Cell 1994; 79: 315–328.
5. Sage EH. Pieces of 8 – bioactive fragments of extracellular proteins as regulators of angiogenesis. Trends Cell Biol 1997; 7: 182–186.
6. Oberbauer R. Not nonsense but antisense – applications of antisense oligonucleotides in different fields of medicine. Wien Klin Wochenschr 1997; 109: 40–46.

CHAPTER 22

1. Shaw PJ. Science, medicine, and the future. Brit med J 1999; 318: 1118–1121.
2. Strong MJ, Grace GM, Orange JB, Leeper HA. Cognition, language, and speech in amyotrophic lateral sclerosis: a review. J Clin Exp Neuropsychol 1996; 18: 291–303.
3. Kurtzke JF. Epidemiology of amyotrophic lateral sclerosis. Adv Neurol 1982; 36: 281–302.
4. Riggs JE. Trauma, axonal injury, and amyotrophic lateral sclerosis: a clinical correlate of a neuropharmacologic model. Clin Neuropharmacol 1995; 18: 273–276.
5. Rowland LP. Controversies about amyotrophic lateral sclerosis. Neurologia 1996; 11(Suppl 5): 72–74.
6. Longstreth WT, Nelson LM, Koepsell TD, van Belle G. Hypotheses to explain the association between vigorous physical activity and amyotrophic lateral sclerosis. Med Hypotheses 1991; 34: 144–148.
7. Mizusawa H, Nakamura H, Wakayama I, et al. Skein-like inclusions in the anterior horn cells in motor neuron disease. J Neurol Sci 1991; 105: 14–21.
8. Delisle MB, Carpenter S. Neurofibrillary axonal swellings and amyotrophic lateral sclerosis. J Neurol Sci 1984; 63: 241–250.

9. Migheli A, Attanasio A, Schiffer D. Ubiquitin and neurofilament expression in anterior horn cells in amyotrophic lateral sclerosis: possible clues to the pathogenesis. Neuropathol Appl Neurobiol 1994; 20: 282–289.
10. Leigh PN, Whitwell H, Garofalo O, et al. Ubiquitin-immunoreactive intraneuronal inclusions in amyotrophic lateral sclerosis. Morphology, distribution, and specificity. Brain 1991; 114: 775–788.
11. Galvin JE, Lee VM, Baba M, et al. Monoclonal antibodies to purified cortical Lewy bodies recognize the mid-size neurofilament subunit. Ann Neurol 1997; 42: 595–603.
12. Sasaki S, Maruyama S. Immunocytochemical and ultrastructural studies of hyaline inclusions in sporadic motor neuron disease. Acta Neuropathol(Berl) 1991; 82: 295–301.
13. Okamoto K, Hirai S, Amari M, et al. Bunina bodies in amyotrophic lateral sclerosis immunostained with rabbit anti-cystatin C serum. Neurosci Lett 1993; 162: 125–128.
14. Kasarskis EJ, Tandon L, Lovell MA, et al. Aluminum, calcium, and iron in the spinal cord of patients with sporadic amyotrophic lateral sclerosis using laser microprobe mass spectroscopy: a preliminary study. J Neurol Sci 1995; 130: 203–208.
15. Davies SW, Turmaine M, Cozens BA, et al. Formation of neuronal intranuclear inclusions underlies the neurological dysfunction in mice transgenic for the HD mutation. Cell 1997; 90: 537–548.
16. Scherzinger E, Lurz R, Turmaine M, et al. Huntingtin-encoded polyglutamine expansions form amyloid-like protein aggregates in vitro and in vivo. Cell 1997; 90: 549–558.
17. Yoshida S, Mitani K, Wakayama I, et al. Bunina body formation in amyotrophic lateral sclerosis: a morphometric-statistical and trace element study featuring aluminum. J Neurol Sci 1995; 130: 88–94.
18. Takahashi H, Ohama E, Ikuta F. Are bunina bodies of endoplasmic reticulum origin? An ultrastructural study of subthalamic eosinophilic inclusions in a case of atypical motor neuron disease. Acta Pathol Jpn 1991; 41: 889–894.
19. Shaw PJ, Ince PG, Falkous G, et al. Cytoplasmic, lysosomal and matrix protease activities in spinal cord tissue from amyotrophic lateral sclerosis (ALS) and control patients. J Neurol Sci 1996; 139(Suppl): 71–75.
20. Martin LJ, Al-Abdulla NA, Brambrink AM, et al. Neurodegeneration in excitotoxicity, global cerebral ischemia, and target deprivation: A perspective on the contributions of apoptosis and necrosis. Brain Res Bull 1998; 46: 281–309.
21. Mu X, He J, Anderson DW, Trojanowski JQ, Springer JE. Altered expression of bcl-2 and bax mRNA in amyotrophic lateral sclerosis spinal cord motor neurons. Ann Neurol 1996; 40: 379–386.
22. Lotz M, Setareh M, von Kempis J, Schwarz H. The nerve growth factor/tumor necrosis factor receptor family. J Leukoc Biol 1996; 60: 1–7.
23. Tandan R, Bradley WG. Amyotrophic lateral sclerosis: Part 2. Etiopathogenesis. Ann Neurol 1985; 18: 419–431.

24. Su M, Wakabayashi K, Tanno Y, et al. An autopsy case of amyotrophic lateral sclerosis with concomitant Alzheimer's and incidental Lewy body diseases [Japanese]. No To Shinkei 1996; 48: 931–936.
25. Williams LR. Oxidative stress, age-related neurodegeneration, and the potential for neurotrophic treatment. Cerebrovasc Brain Metab Rev 1995; 7: 55–73.
26. Gorman AM, McGowan A, O'Neill C, Cotter T. Oxidative stress and apoptosis in neurodegeneration. J Neurol Sci 1996; 139(Suppl): 45–52.
27. Cooper B. The epidemiology of primary degenerative dementia and related neurological disorders. Eur Arch Psychiatry Clin Neurosci 1991; 240: 223–233.
28. Eki T, Abe M, Furuya K, et al. A long-range physical map of human chromosome 21q22.1 band from the YAC continuum. Mamm Genome 1996; 7: 303–311.
29. Andersen PM, Forsgren L, Binzer M, et al. Autosomal recessive adult-onset amyotrophic lateral sclerosis associated with homozygosity for Asp90Ala CuZn-superoxide dismutase mutation. A clinical and genealogical study of 36 patients. Brain 1996; 119: 1153–1172.
30. Lyons TJ, Liu H, Goto JJ, et al. Mutations in copper-zinc superoxide dismutase that cause amyotrophic lateral sclerosis alter the zinc binding site and the redox behavior of the protein. Proc Natl Acad Sci USA 1996; 93: 12240–12244.
31. Cote F, Collard JF, Julien JP. Progressive neuronopathy in transgenic mice expressing the human neurofilament heavy gene: a mouse model of amyotrophic lateral sclerosis. Cell 1993; 73: 35–46.
32. Price DL, Koliatsos VE, Wong PC, et al. Motor neuron disease and model systems: aetiologies, mechanisms and therapies. Ciba Found Symp 1996; 196: 3–13.
33. Siddique T, Deng HX. Genetics of amyotrophic lateral sclerosis. Hum Mol Genet 1996; 5(Spec No): 1465–1470.
34. Przedborski S, Donaldson D, Jakowec M, et al. Brain superoxide dismutase, catalase, and glutathione peroxidase activities in amyotrophic lateral sclerosis. Ann Neurol 1996; 39: 158–165.
35. Cummings JF, de Lahunta A, Summers BA, et al. Eosinophilic cytoplasmic inclusions in sporadic equine motor neuron disease: an electron microscopic study . Acta Neuropathol(Berl) 1993; 85: 291–297.
36. de la Rua-Domenech R, Wiedmann M, Mohammed HO, et al. Equine motor neuron disease is not linked to Cu/Zn superoxide dismutase mutations: sequence analysis of the equine Cu/Zn superoxide dismutase cDNA. Gene 1996; 178: 83–88.
37. Shaw PJ, Tomkins J, Slade JY, et al. CNS tissue Cu/Zn superoxide dismutase (SOD1) mutations in motor neurone disease (MND). Neuroreport 1997; 8: 3923–3927.
38. Shaw IC, Fitzmaurice PS, Mitchell JD, Lynch PG. Studies on cellular free radical protection mechanisms in the anterior horn from patients with amyotrophic lateral sclerosis. Neurodegeneration 1995; 4: 391–396.

39. Oyanagi K, Makifuchi T, Ohtoh T, et al. Amyotrophic lateral sclerosis of Guam: the nature of the neuropathological findings. Acta Neuropathol (Berl) 1994; 88: 405–412.
40. Troost D, van den Oord JJ, de Jong JM, Swaab DF. Lymphocytic infiltration in the spinal cord of patients with amyotrophic lateral sclerosis. Clin Neuropathol 1989; 8: 289–294.
41. Smith RG, Engelhardt JI, Tajti J, Appel SH. Experimental immune-mediated motor neuron diseases: models for human ALS. Brain Res Bull 1993; 30: 373–380.
42. Appel SH, Smith RG, Engelhardt JI, Stefani E. Evidence for autoimmunity in amyotrophic lateral sclerosis. J Neurol Sci 1994; 124(Suppl): 14–19.
43. Werdelin L, Boysen G, Jensen TS, Mogensen P. Immunosuppressive treatment of patients with amyotrophic lateral sclerosis. Acta Neurol Scand 1990; 82: 132–134.
44. Jaspert A, Claus D, Grehl H, Neundorfer B. Multifocal motor neuropathy: clinical and electrophysiological findings. J Neurol 1996; 243: 684–692.
45. Swanson NR, Fox SA, Mastaglia FL. Search for persistent infection with poliovirus or other enteroviruses in amyotrophic lateral sclerosis-motor neurone disease. Neuromuscul Disord 1995; 5: 457–465.
46. Muller WK, Schaltenbrand G. Attempts to reproduce amyotrophic lateral sclerosis in laboratory animals by inoculation of Schu virus isolated from a patient with apparent amyotrophic lateral sclerosis. J Neurol 1979; 220: 1–19.
47. Gardner MB, Rasheed S, Klement V, et al. Lower motor neuron disease in wild mice caused by indigenous type C virus and search for a similar etiology in human amyotrophic lateral sclerosis. UCLA Forum Med Sci 1976; 217–234.
48. Kennedy PG. On the possible role of viruses in the aetiology of motor neurone disease: a review. J R Soc Med 1990; 83: 784–787.
49. Hughes RA, O'Leary PD. Neurotrophic factors and the development of drugs to promote motoneuron survival. Clin Exp Pharmacol Physiol 1996; 23: 965–969.
50. Ono S, Imai T, Shimizu N, et al. Ciliary neurotropic factor in skin biopsies of patients with amyotrophic lateral sclerosis. Lancet 1998; 352: 958–959.
51. Pamphlett R, Waley P. Motor neuron uptake of low dose inorganic mercury. J Neurol Sci 1996; 135: 63–67.
52. Perl DP. Relationship of aluminum to Alzheimer's disease. Environ Health Perspect 1985; 63: 149–153.
53. Plato CC, Garruto RM, Fox KM, Gajdusek DC. Amyotrophic lateral sclerosis and parkinsonism-dementia on Guam: a 25-year prospective case-control study. Am J Epidemiol 1986; 124: 643–656.
54. Kalfakis N, Vassilopoulos D, Voumvourakis C, et al. Amyotrophic lateral sclerosis in southern Greece: an epidemiologic study. Neuroepidemiology 1991; 10: 170–173.

55. Tosi L, Righetti C, Adami L, Zanette G. October 1942: a strange epidemic paralysis in Saval, Verona, Italy. Revision and diagnosis 50 years later of tri-ortho-cresyl phosphate poisoning. J Neurol Neurosurg Psychiatry 1994; 57: 810–813.

56. Hansen JC, Danscher G. Organic mercury: an environmental threat to the health of dietary-exposed societies? Rev Environ Health 1997; 12: 107–116.

57. Nagashima K. A review of experimental methylmercury toxicity in rats: neuropathology and evidence for apoptosis. Toxicol Pathol 1997; 25: 624–631.

58. Calne DB, Peppard RF. Aging of the nigrostriatal pathway in humans. Can J Neurol Sci 1987; 14: 424–427.

59. Shaw PJ. Excitotoxicity and motor neurone disease: a review of the evidence. J Neurol Sci 1994; 124(Suppl): 6–13.

60. Siklos L, Engelhardt J, Harati Y, et al. Ultrastructural evidence for altered calcium in motor nerve terminals in amyotropic lateral sclerosis. Ann Neurol 1996; 39: 203–216.

61. Hatazawa J, Brooks RA, Dalakas MC, et al. Cortical motor-sensory hypometabolism in amyotrophic lateral sclerosis: a PET study. J Comput Assist Tomogr 1988; 12: 630–636.

62. Waldemar G, Vorstrup S, Jensen TS, et al. Focal reductions of cerebral blood flow in amyotrophic lateral sclerosis: a [99mTc]-d,l-HMPAO SPECT study. J Neurol Sci 1992; 107: 19–28.

63. Kew JJ, Leigh PN, Playford ED, et al. Cortical function in amyotrophic lateral sclerosis. A positron emission tomography study. Brain 1993; 116: 655–680.

64. Talbot PR, Goulding PJ, Lloyd JJ, et al. Inter-relation between "classic" motor neuron disease and frontotemporal dementia: neuropsychological and single photon emission computed tomography study. J Neurol Neurosurg Psychiatry 1995; 58: 541–547.

65. Bensimon G, Lacomblez L, Meininger V. A controlled trial of riluzole in amyotrophic lateral sclerosis. ALS/Riluzole Study Group. N Engl J Med 1994; 330: 585–591.

66. Hirayama B, Hazama A, Loo DF, et al. Transport of cycasin by the intestinal Na+/glucose cotransporter. Biochim Biophys Acta 1994; 1193: 151–154.

67. Dickinson CJ. Cerebral oxidative metabolism in essential hypertension: A meta-analysis. J Hypertension 1995; 13: 653–658.

68. Harno K, Rissanen A, Palo J. Glucose tolerance in amyotrophic lateral sclerosis. Acta Neurol Scand 1984; 70: 451–455.

69. Dalakas MC, Hatazawa J, Brooks RA, Di Chiro G. Lowered cerebral glucose utilization in amyotrophic lateral sclerosis. Ann Neurol 1987; 22: 580–586.

70. Mathe JF, Feve JR, Labat JJ, et al. Ischemia of the anterior horn of the spinal cord [French]. Rev Neurol(Paris) 1989; 145: 60–64.

71. Fraser H, Behan W, Chree A, et al. Mouse inoculation studies reveal no

transmissible agent in amyotrophic lateral sclerosis. Brain Pathol 1996; 6: 89–99.

72. Horwich AL, Weissman JS. Deadly conformations – protein misfolding in prion disease. Cell 1997; 89: 499–510.

73. Bruijn LI, Becher MW, Lee MK, et al. ALS-linked SOD1 mutant G85R mediates damage to astrocytes and promotes rapidly progressive disease with SOD1-containing inclusions. Neuron 1997; 18: 327–338.

74. Craig EA, Gambill BD, Nelson RJ. Heat shock proteins: molecular chaperones of protein biogenesis. Microbiol Rev 1993; 57: 402–414.

75. Martin J, Hartl FU. Chaperone-assisted protein folding. Curr Opin Struct Biol 1997; 7: 41–52.

76. Melnick J, Argon Y. Molecular chaperones and the biosynthesis of antigen receptors. Immunol Today 1995; 16: 243–250.

77. Tomkins J, Usher P, Slade JY, et al. Novel insertion in the KSP region of the neurofilament heavy gene in amyotrophic lateral sclerosis (ALS). Neuroreport 1998; 9: 3967–3970.

78. Saper CB, Wainer BH, German DC. Axonal and transneuronal transport in the transmission of neurological disease: potential role in system degenerations, including Alzheimer's disease. Neuroscience 1987; 23: 389–398.

79. Wong PC, Borchelt DR. Motor neuron disease caused by mutations in superoxide dismutase 1. Curr Opin Neurol 1995; 8: 294–301.

80. Linnane AW, Marzuki S, Ozawa T, Tanaka M. Mitochondrial DNA mutations as an important contributor to ageing and degenerative diseases. Lancet 1989; i: 642–645.

81. Beal MF. Aging, energy, and oxidative stress in neurodegenerative diseases. Ann Neurol 1995; 38: 357–366.

82. Cann RL, Stoneking M, Wilson AC. Mitochondrial DNA and human evolution. Nature 1987; 325: 31–36.

83. Yase Y. Amyotrophic lateral sclerosis – causative role of trace elements [Japanese]. Nippon Rinsho 1996; 54: 123–128.

84. Rothstein JD, Kuncl RW. Neuroprotective strategies in a model of chronic glutamate-mediated motor neuron toxicity. J Neurochem 1995; 65: 643–651.

85. Virgo L, de Belleroche J. Induction of the immediate early gene c-jun in human spinal cord in amyotrophic lateral sclerosis with concomitant loss of NMDA receptor NR-1 and glycine transporter mRNA. Brain Res 1995; 676: 196–204.

86. Smith MD, Dawson SJ, Latchman DS. The Brn-3a transcription factor induces neuronal process outgrowth and the coordinate expression of genes encoding synaptic proteins. Mol Cell Biol 1997; 17: 345–354.

INDEX

retinal arteries 136, 189
retrograde menstruation 103
retroviruses 26, 76
rheumatoid, arthritis 71, 192
ribosenucleic acid (RNA) 205
rickettsial infections 114
riluzole 224
rotavirus 50

salicylic acid 46
salmonella infections 53
scale, skin 43
schizophrenia and arthritis 71
sclerosis, multiple, *see* multiple sclerosis
serotonin 55, 137, 182
    antagonists, in migraine 134
sexual intercourse 110, 174
sheep, bad teeth in 98
single photon emission computerised
    tomography (SPECT) 81, 118
SLE 74
sleep, bowel function effects 54
smoking effects, Alzheimer's disease 84
    inflammatory bowel disease 125
    pulmonary hypertension 182
    rheumatoid arthritis 71
sodium 159
SPECT imaging of brain 81, 118
sperms 104, 175
sphygmomanometer 143
spinal cord, sub-acute combined
    degeneration 197, 200
spontaneous hypertensive rat 156
staphylococci, in psoriasis 46
    infections 192
steroids, in asthma 7, 11
    in psoriasis 44
    in vasculitides 189
streptococci, in psoriasis 46
strokes, in hypertension 157
sulfathalazine 127, 130
sumatriptan 134
superantigens 46
superoxide dismutase 218, 135
sympathetic nervous system 11, 155, 166,
    173
syncope, *see* fainting
synovium 71
systemic lupus erythematosus (SLE) 74,
    169
systolic arterial pressure 144

tacrine 88
Takayasu's disease 187
tampon use and endometriosis 105
tar preparations 46
tau proteins 86
T-cells, *see* lymphocytes
telomerase 205
telomeres 205
temporal arteritis 188
TNFα 43
temporal arteritis 188
temporal lobe, of brain 81
thromboxane 172
togavirus 221
tracking, of blood pressure 156
transforming growth factor-beta 63
transplantation, heart 36
triplet-repeats 216
triptans 134
Tropheryma whippelii 96
tuberculous infection 129
tumour necrosis factor 43, 74, 128, 173,
    217

ubiquitin 82, 215
ulcerative colitis 123
upper motor neurones 22
urine volume 159

vagus nerves 32, 38
vascular endothelial growth factor
    (VEGF) 207, 175
vasculitis 187, 191
vasopressin 155
veins, constriction 33
ventricles, cardiac 143
    septal defect 180
vertebral arteries 152
viruses 25, 52, 94, 114, 221
vitamins 195
    B2 complex 195
    B12 deficiency 198

Wegener's granulomatosis 190, 192
wheezing, in asthma 8
Whipple's disease 96
worm infestation 12, 117

yeasts, in psoriasis 46

zolmitriptan 134